MW00849509

# The Essence of

# Kriya Yoga

## By
## Paramhansa Yogananda

Alight Publications
2006

# The Essence of Kriya Yoga

**By Paramhansa Yogananda**

First Edition Published in January, 2006

Alight Publications
PO Box 930
Union City, CA 94587
*http://www.alightbooks.com*

ISBN 1-931833-18-4

Printed in the United States of America

Dedicated
to
Sincere Seekers
of
the Way

# Contents

**The Essence of Kriya Yoga**

# Introduction

By the grace of Shiva-Goraksha-Babaji, Mukunda Lal Ghosh was born in the northern Indian town of Gorakhpur on January 5th, 1893. Gorakhpur is one of the main centers dedicated to the worship of the Mahavatar Babaji who has guided the spiritual evolution of humanity for eons. Mukunda was to later become the world renowned yogi, Paramhansa Yogananda, whose life-work was to introduce true spirituality to the West. He was the bridge between the East and the West.

Although widely respected and venerated, his true work is still not fully recognized. The immensity of what he achieved in his lifetime may never be truly known. His skillful means of transmitting alien concepts and difficult practices through innovative methods that had not been used before is unprecedented. His influence on many spiritual movements in the West is unheralded.

We can only pay our humble homage to such a selfless Master in the silence of our hearts, in the bliss of our meditations, and in the roar of Om.

Born into a devout and well-to-do Bengali family, Yogananda was encouraged to pursue his own spiritual path at an early age. By age 11, he was having mystical experiences, and, in one such episode in 1904, his mother, who was traveling away from home at the time, appeared to him in a vision. The vision informed him of her imminent death before anyone else in the home even knew that she was ill, and she died just as he had foreseen. His mother had left him a message prior to her death, informing him of his destiny and leaving him an amulet, which opened him to the guidance of teachers from past lives.

Yogananda was then impelled to visit sages and saints, even fleeing home and school occasionally, in a burning desire to find his Guru whose face had appeared to him in a vision. His quest finally led him to Swami Sri Yukteswar, the pre-eminent Master of Kriya Yoga, in 1910, and, for the next ten years, he studied under this master's loving discipline. After graduating from Calcutta University in July 1915, he vowed to devote his life to the love and service of God. He received the name Yogananda, meaning bliss (ananda) through union with the Divine (yoga) when he was initiated into the monastic Swami Order, by his Guru.

Thus began his tireless work to promulgate the teachings of the deathless Babaji, who had initiated Lahiri Mahasaya into Kriya Yoga. In turn Lahiri Mahasaya had passed on his teachings to others, including Sri Yukteswar. One of the distinctive marks of Kriya Yoga was that it was well-suited to the life-style of a householder, and brought the goal of Self-realization to the reach of the ordinary person with a family and responsibilities. The myth that only by renouncing one's family could a spiritual seeker attain to final liberation had been exploded by these Kriya Masters, who had families and lived their lives in awareness and God-attunement without sacrificing their responsibilities. These spiritual giants discharged their duties without attachment.

In 1917, Yogananda founded a school for boys that combined yoga training and spiritual instruction with modern educational methods. He joked in his autobiography that, after having renounced family life (for the sake of l his ife-work to spread spirituality in the West), he became father to more boys than he ever would otherwise have had.

A pivotal point came, when Babaji instructed Sri Yukteswar to prepare Yogananda for the great task for which he'd been born, the spiritualization of the Western World. In 1920, Yogananda was appointed to be one of the international delegates to a congress of religious leaders to be held in Boston. He knew nobody in the United States, and nobody knew anything of him. But that would change rapidly.

Yoganandaji's maiden address in Boston, on **"The Science of Religion,"** exploring the common threads between the world's religions, was enthusiastically received. For the next several years, he lectured and taught on the East coast of the United States, and in 1924 he embarked on a cross-continental speaking tour. He started a two-month series of lectures and classes in Los Angeles in January of 1925. As elsewhere, his talks were greeted with interest and acclaim. The Los Angeles Times reported: "The Philharmonic Auditorium presents the extraordinary spectacle of thousands…being turned away an hour before the advertised opening of a lecture with the 3000-seat hall filled to its utmost capacity."

During the next decade his work and spirit brought him many famous students, including Luther Burbank, George Eastman, and Leopold Stokowski. In 1927, Yogananda was invited to meet President Calvin Coolidge at the White House. In less than a century, he would be hailed as the father of yoga in the West for his pioneering role in making known India's ancient philosophy of yoga and its time-honored tradition of meditation.

Yogananda's arrival in America from India initiated an upsurge of interest in the spiritual wisdom of the East. Through his life and teachings, he made an indelible impression on the spiritual landscape of the United States and the world. "Yogananda has become an image — a remarkable, deep, sweet, poetic, ecstatic man enraptured of cosmic life — who has changed the map of American religious life," writes Robert S. Ellwood, Ph.D., the former chairman of University of Southern California's School of Religion.

This "Hindoo Holy Man" as the headlines of the day called him, has great influence to this day though his best-selling life story, the classic **Autobiography of a Yogi**, which was published in 1946 and expanded by him in subsequent editions. In 1999 the book was named one of the one hundred most influential spiritual books of the twentieth century. Phyllis Tickle, a contributing editor to *Publishers Weekly* noted, "Few books ... have had greater impact on popular theology than Paramahansa Yogananda's

*Autobiography of a Yogi."* In *A New Religious America,* noted Harvard University Professor of Comparative Religions Diana Eck writes, "Yogananda put yoga on the map in America."

He stayed in the United States for the better part of three decades, introducing the principles of yoga and the art of balanced spiritual living to hundreds of thousands of people through his extensive public lecture tours, his numerous writings, and the centers he founded in the United States, Canada, and abroad.

In 1935, Yogananda began an 18-month tour of Europe and India during which he met statesmen, scientists, and spiritual figures. That year, his guru, Sri Yukteswar, bestowed on him the title Paramhansa[1] (meaning "supreme swan") recognizing his role as a World Teacher and great Soul.

India's great political and moral leader, Mahatma Gandhi invited Yogananda to his Wardha ashram. At Gandhiji's request he initiated the Mahatma and a few satyagrahis (followers of truth action with non-violence) into the liberating technique of Kriya Yoga.

At about 7:00 PM on March 9, 1936, Yogananda's beloved guru, consciously entered into a supreme God communion state and through off his mortal coils. A few months later, on June 19, while Yoganandaji was meditating, a beautiful light appeared before him. It was Sri Yukteswar in his resurrected body to reveal through speech as well as through thought transference the laws of the universe and other esoteric matters. It is interesting to note that an image of Sri Yukteswar can be found on the cover art of the Beatles widely acclaimed "Sgt. Pepper's Lonely Heart's Club Band" album!

Yogananda's own physical death came on March 7, 1952, a conscious exit made after a speech given at a banquet. Twenty days later, according to a signed and notarized statement from the director of Forest Lawn Memorial Park, "no physical disintegration was visited upon his body…it was apparently in a phenomenal state of immutability." Yogananda's passing received widespread coverage in the press, including *The New York Times,* the *Los Angeles Times,* and *Time* magazine. In 1977, on the occasion of the 25th anniversary of Yogananda's passing, the government of India formally recognized his outstanding contributions to the spiritual upliftment of humanity by issuing a commemorative stamp in his honor, together with a tribute that read, in part:

"The ideal of love for God and service to humanity found full expression in the life of Paramahansa Yogananda. ... Though the major part of his life was spent outside India, still, [he] takes his place among our great saints. His work continues to grow and shine ever more brightly, drawing people everywhere on the path of the pilgrimage of the Spirit."

Yogananda's best-known written works include his **Autobiography of a Yogi**, published in 1946. Since its initial release, this book has been in continuous publication and translated into 18 languages. Through his writings he has been able to disseminate to a wide international audience his belief in the unity of the world's religions and to teach his methods for attaining direct personal experience of God. To serious students he taught Kriya yoga, a spiritual science including soul-awakening techniques that had been lost in the Dark Ages but revived by his Guru lineage.

Yogananda took every opportunity to foster interfaith understanding, brotherhood, and world peace. Just a sampling of his myriad efforts in this area include: speaking at a World Peace Meeting in Boston, 1922; speaking at a conference on interracial relations in New York, 1929; addressing the World Fellowship of Faiths at the Chicago World's Fair, 1933; speaking at the British National Council of World Fellowship of Faiths at Whitefields Institute in England, 1936; hosting an International Peace Program in Los Angeles, 1939; and addressing an international peace conference (which he helped organize) held in San Francisco during the inaugural meetings of the United Nations, 1945.

"If we had a man like Paramahansa Yogananda in the United Nations today," said Dr. Binay R. Sen, former Indian ambassador to the United States, "probably the world would be a better place than it is."

In this new millennium, Yogananda's message is still relevant and just as needed. Global events continue to challenge people throughout the world to look at life from a deeper spiritual perspective, to seek a sense of inner peace and security that can withstand the changing winds of outer circumstances, and to discover the shared values that unify humanity, while acknowledging cultural and religious diversity. The core of Yogananda's mission addressed these very concerns, and his spiritual teachings provide answers as relevant to seekers today as when he began his mission more than eighty-six years ago.

The core of Yogananda's work involved Kriya Yoga. Although the actual practice of Kriya Yoga is not given in books to the public to ensure its proper and beneficial transmission, his whole life, speeches and writings give the Essence of Kriya Yoga.

I've chosen to provide to the reader a selection which I personally consider to be most helpful for all spiritual seekers, and especially to those who practice some form of Kriya Yoga.

This volume consists of the 4th edition (1925) of **The Science of Religion**. This forms the basic foundation for all yogic practice. Yoga is not a religion, but the science of Self-Realization and Self-Actualization. When the common factors of the great religions are contemplated, shorn of non-essentials, an understanding bridging all faiths, cultures and times can be accomplished.

In his **Songs of the Soul**, Yogananda , through the medium of his poems allows us a rare glimpse into the relationship between a Self-realized soul, one who has mastered the art and science of yoga, and the goal of Yoga, the Divine Beloved. The poems are from the 3rd enlarged Edition of 1925.

In order to bring Yoga into our lives, we need to examine our life-style. One of the main elements which Yogananda always stressed was diet and health. A selection of his writings on **Fasting and Diets,** as well as a few recipes, are given for reference. Yogananda was a keen cook, and would on occasion cook for his disciples!

The essence of Kriya Yoga can be best understood through Yogananda's experiences with his Guru, Sri Yukteswar. A selection from the masterful **Autobiography of a Yogi,** gives all the chapters which reveals these hidden teachings. They are all from the 1946 1st edition.

A lasting contribution is the introduction of the Immortal Babaji, and any understanding of Yoga as Spiritual Evolution requires a homage to this Divine Being.

An excerpt from an article written by Yoganandaji in the March 1937 issue of Inner Culture, called, "Yogavatar Shama Lahiri Mahasaya's Ladder." is also provided as it sheds important light on the system of Kriya Yoga and the Second Coming of Christ.

May this compilation provide the reader with a source of inspiration and connection to Paramhansa Yogananda, whose presence still permeates our world.

Runbir Singh
Editor
January 5th, 2006

---

[1] Yoganandaji spelled some Sanskrit Indian words according to how they would be pronounced rather than how they were supposed to be written according to scholarly systems (primarily formulated by Western scholars, not too familiar with the living language). This was the case with his title of "Paramhansa" which he wrote in the latter manner, rather than the more formal "Paramahansa."

Kriya Yoga, the scientific technique of God-realization will ultimately spread in all lands, and aid in harmonizing the nations through man's personal, transcendental perception of the Infinite Father

Babaji

Divine Union is possible through self-effort and is not dependent on theological beliefs or on the arbitrary will of a Cosmic Dictator.

Lahiri Mahasaya

# The Science of Religion

## CHAPTER 1
### INTRODUCTION

The purpose of this book is to outline what should be understood by religion, in order to make it universally and pragmatically necessary. It also seeks to present that aspect of the idea of the God-head which has a direct bearing on the motives and actions of every minute of our lives. It is true that God is Infinite in His nature and aspects, and it is also true that to prepare a chart detailing, so far as is consistent with reason, what God is like is only an evidence of the limitations of the human mind in its attempt to fathom God. Still, it is equally true that the human mind, in spite of all its drawbacks, cannot rest perfectly satisfied with what is finite. It has a natural urge to interpret what is human and finite in the light of what is super-human and infinite-what it feels but cannot express, what within it lies implicit but under circumstances refuses to be explicit.

Our ordinary conception of God is that He is Super-human, Infinite, Omnipresent, Omniscient, and the like. In this general conception there are many variations. Some call God Personal, some Impersonal, and so forth. The point emphasized in this book is that whatever conception we have of God, if it does not influence our daily conduct, if everyday life does not find an inspiration from it, and if it is not found universally necessary, then that conception is useless. If God is not conceived in such a way that we cannot do without Him in the satisfaction of a want, in our dealings with people, in earning money, in reading a book, in passing an examination, in the doing of the most trifling or the highest duties, then it is plain that we have not felt any connection between God and life. God may be Infinite, Omnipresent, Omniscient, Personal and Merciful, but these conceptions are not sufficiently compelling to make us try to know God. We may as well do without Him. He may be Infinite, Omnipresent, and so forth, but we have no immediate and practical use for those conceptions in our busy, rushing lives.

We fall back on those conceptions only when we seek to justify, in philosophical and poetical writings, in art or in idealistic talks, the finite craving for something beyond; when we, with all our vaunted knowledge, are at a loss to explain some of the most common phenomena of the universe; or when we get stranded in the vicissitudes of the world. "We pray to the Ever-Merciful when we get stuck," as the Eastern maxim has it. Otherwise, we seem to get along all right in our work-a-day world without Him. These stereotyped conceptions appear to be the safety-valves of our pent-up human thought. They explain Him, but do not make us seek Him. They lack motive power. We are not necessarily seeking God when we call Him Infinite, Omnipresent, All-Merciful, and so forth. These conceptions satisfy the intellect, but do not soothe the soul. If respected and cherished in our hearts, they may broaden us to a certain extent-may make us moral and resigned toward Him. But they do not make God our own-they are not intimate enough. They place Him aloof from everyday concerns of the world.

These conceptions savor of outlandishness when we are on the street, in a factory, behind a counter, or in an office. Not because we are really dead to God and religion, but because we lack a proper conception of them – a conception that can be interwoven with the fabric of daily life. What we conceive of God should be of daily, nay hourly, guidance to us. The very conception of God should stir us to seek Him in the midst of our daily and compelling conception of God. We should take religion and God out of the sphere of belief into that of daily life. If we do not emphasize the necessity of God in every aspect of our lives and the need of religion in every minute of our existence, then God and religion drop out of our intimate daily consideration and become only a one-day-in-a-week affair. In the next chapter of this work an attempt is made to show that *in order to understand the real necessity of God and religion we muse throw emphasis on that conception of both which is most relevant to the chief aim of our daily and hourly actions.*

This book also aims to point out the universality and unity of religion. There have been different religions in different ages. There have been heated controversy, long warfare, and much bloodshed over them. One religion has stood against an other, one sect has fought with another. Not only is there a variety in religions, but there is also a wide diversity of sects and opinions within the same religion. But the question arises, when there is one God, why there should be so many religions?

It may be argued that particular stages of intellectual growth and special types of mentality belonging to certain nations, owing to different geographical locations and other extraneous circumstances, determine the origin of different religions, such as Hinduism, Mohammedanism and Buddhism, for the Asiatics, Christianity for the Westerners and so forth. If by religion we understand only practices, particular tenets, dogmas, customs and conventions, then there may be ground for the existence of so many religions; but if religion means, *primarily*, God-consciousness, or the realization of god both within and without; *secondarily* a body of beliefs, tenets, and dogmas, the, strictly speaking, there is but one religion in the world, for there is but one religion in the world, for there is but one God. The different customs, forms of worship, tenets, and conventions may be held to form the grounds for the origin of different denominations and sects included under that one religion. If religion is understood in this way, then and then only can its universality be maintained, for we can not possibly universalize particular customs or conventions. Only the element common to all religions can be universalized. We can ask every one to follow that. Then can it be truly said that religion is not only necessary but it is universal, as well. Everyone must follow the same religion, for there is but one, its universal element being one and the same. Only its customs and conventions differ.

I have tried to show in this book that *as God is one, necessary for all of us, so Religion is one, necessary and universal.* Only the roads to it may differ in some respects at the beginning. As a matter of fact, it is ludicrous to say that there are two religions, when there is but one God. There may be two denominations or sects, but there is only one religion. What we now call different religions should be known as different denominations or sects under that one universal religion. And what we now know as different denominations or sects should be specified as different branch cults or creeds. If we once know the meaning of the word "religion," which I am going to discuss presently, we shall naturally be very circumspect in the use of it. It is only the limited human point of view that overlooks the underlying universal element in the so called different religions of the world, and this overlooking has been the cause of many evils.

This book gives a psychological definition of religion, not an objective definition based on dogmas or tenets. In other words, it seeks to make religion a question of our whole inward being and attitude, and not a mere observance of certain rules and precepts, not an intellectual acquiescence, either, in certain beliefs about God, the universe, and so forth. On this psychological ground its universality has been established. I have also discussed the merits and demerits of the different methods for the attainment of that religious consciousness which is here set forth.

It should always be remembered that when the theory and practice of religion are poles apart, we must not stop at the theory and lose energy over comment or criticism thereon, leaving out of sight the practical aspect of it that alone can lead to its true understanding. The verification of a theory lies in practice. If a practice truly followed is found at last to militate against the theory, then, and not till then, may the theory be safely rejected.

## CHAPTER II
THE UNIVERSALITY, NECESSITY, AND ONENESS OF RELIGION;
THE DISTINCTION BETWEEN PLEASURE, PAIN, AND BLISS: GOD

First we must know what religion is, then only can we judge whether it is necessary for all of us to be religious.

Without necessity there is no action. Every action of ours has an end of its own for which we perform it. People of the world act variously to accomplish various ends. There is a multiplicity of ends determining the actions of men in the world.

But is there any common and universal end of all the actions of all the people of the world? Is there *any common, highest necessity* for all of us which prompts us to all actions? A little analysis of the motives and ends of men's actions in the world shows that, though there are a thousand and one proximate or immediate ends of men in regard to the particular calling or profession which they take up, the ultimate end-which all other ends merely subserve – is the avoidance of pain and want, and the attainment of permanent Bliss. Whether we can at all permanently avoid pain and want, and obtain Bliss, is a separate question, but as a matter of fact, in all our actions, we obviously try to avoid the former and reach the latter.

Why does a man serve as an apprentice? Because he wishes to become an expert in a certain business. Why does he engage in that particular business? Because money can be earned therein. Why should money be earned at all? Because it will satisfy personal and family wants. Why must wants be fulfilled? Because pain will thereby be removed and Bliss be gained.

As a matter of fact, happiness and Bliss are not the same thing. We all aim at Bliss, but through a great blunder we imagine pleasure and happiness to be Bliss. How that has come to be so will be shown presently. The ultimate motive is really Bliss, which we feel inwardly; but happiness – or pleasure- has taken its place, through our misunderstanding, and the latter has come to be regarded as the ultimate motive.

Thus we see that the fulfillment of some want, removal of some pain, physical or mental, from the slightest to the acutest, and the attainment of Bliss, form our ultimate end. We can not question further why Bliss is to be gained, for no answer can be given. That is our ultimate end, no matter what we do- enter a business, earn money, seek friends, write books, acquire knowledge, rule kingdoms, donate millions, explore countries, look for fame, help the needy, become philanthropists, or embrace martyrdom. And it will be shown that the seeking of God becomes a real fact to us when that end is kept rigorously in view. Millions may be the steps, myriads may be the intermediate acts and motives; but the ultimate motive is always the same- to attain permanent Bliss, even though it be through a long chain of actions.

Man likes to, and has to, go along the chain to get to the final end. He may commit suicide to end some pain, or perpetrate murder to get rid of some form of want or pain or some cruel heart-thrust, thinking he will thereby attain a real satisfaction or relief, which he mistakes for Bliss. But the point to notice is that here, too, is the same working (though wrongly) toward the ultimate end.

Some one may say, "I do not care anything about pleasure or happiness. I live life to accomplish something, to achieve success." Another says: "I want to do good in the world. I do not care whether I am in pain or not." But if you look into the minds of these people you will find that there is the same working toward the goal of happiness. Does the first want a success that has in its achievement no pleasure or happiness? Does the second want to do good to others, yet himself get no happiness in doing it? Obviously not. They may not mind a thousand and one physical pains or mental sufferings inflicted by others, or arising out of situations incidental to the pursuit of success or the doing of good to others; but because the one finds great satisfaction in success, and the other intensely enjoys the happiness of doing good to others, the former seeks success, and the latter others' good, in spite of incidental troubles.

Even the most altruistic motive and the sincerest intention of advancing the good of humanity, for its own sake, have sprung from the basic urge for a chastened personal happiness, approaching Bliss. But it is not the happiness of a narrow self-seeker. It is the happiness of a broad seeker of that "pure self" that is in you and me and all. This happiness is Bliss, a little alloyed. So with Pure Bliss as a personal motive for altruistic action, the altruist is not laying himself open to the charge of narrow selfishness, for one can not himself have Pure Bliss unless he is broad enough to wish and seek it for others, too. That is the universal law.

So if the motives for the actions of all men are traced farther and farther back, the ultimate motive will be found to be the same with all-the removal of pain and the attainment of Bliss. This end being universal, it must be looked upon as the most necessary one. And what is universal and most necessary for man is, of course, religion to him. *Hence religion necessarily consists in the permanent removal of pain and the realization of Bliss or God.* And the actions which we must adopt for the permanent avoidance of pain and the realization of Bliss or God are called religious. If we understand religion in this way, then its universality becomes obvious. For no one can deny that he wants to avoid pain permanently and attain permanent Bliss. This must be universally admitted, since none can gainsay its truth. Man's very existence is bound up with it.

All want to live because they love religion. Even if a man committed suicide it would because he loved religion, too; for by doing that he thinks he will attain a happier state than he finds while living. At any rate, he thinks he will be rid of some pain that is bothering him. In this case his religion is crude. But it is religion, just the same. His goal is perfectly right, the same that all persons have. For all of them want to obtain happiness, or Bliss. But his means are ridiculous. Because of his ignorance he does not know what will bring him to Bliss, the goal of happiness.

Thus, in one sense every one in the world is religious, inasmuch as every one is trying to get rid of want and pain, and gain Bliss. Every one is working for the same goal. But in a strict sense only a few in the world are religious, for only a few in the world, though they have the same goal as all others, know the most effective means for removing, permanently, all pain or want – physical, mental, or spiritual – and gaining true Bliss.

One must bid good-bye to the rigidly narrow orthodox conception of religion, though that conception is, in a remote way, connected with the conception I am bringing out.. If for some time you do not go to church or temple, or attend any of its ceremonies or forms, even though acting religiously in your daily life by being calm, poised, concentrated, charitable, squeezing happiness from the most trying situations, then ordinary people of a pronounced orthodox or narrow bent will nod their heads and declare that, although you are trying to be good, still, from the point of view of religion, or in the eyes of God, you are "falling off," as you did not of late enter the precincts of the holy places.

While of course there cannot be any valid excuse for permanently keeping away from such holy places, there cannot, on the other hand, be any legitimate reason for one's being considered more religious for attending church, if at the same time one neglects to apply in daily life the principles which religion upholds viz, those that make ultimately for the attainment of permanent Bliss. Religion is not dove-tailed with the pews of the church, nor is it bound up with the ceremonies performed therein. If you have an attitude of reverence, if you live your daily life always with a view to bringing undisturbed Bliss-consciousness into it, you will be just as religious out of the church as in it.

Of course this should not be understood as an argument for forsaking the church, which is usually a real help in many ways. The point is that you should put forth just as much effort outside of the church hours to gain eternal happiness as you forego while from the pews you are passively enjoying a good sermon. Not that listening is not a good thing, in its way, for it certainly is.

The word religion is derived from the Latin religare, to bind. What binds, whom does it bind, and why? Leaving aside any orthodox explanation, it stands to reason that it is "we" who are bound. What binds us? Not chains or shackles, of course. Religion may be said to bind us by rules, laws, or injunctions only. And why? To make us slaves? To disallow us the birthright of free thinking or free action? That is unreasonable. Just as religion must have a sufficient motive, so its motive in "binding" us must also be good. What is that motive? The only rational answer we can give is that religion binds us by rules, laws, injunctions, in order that we may not degenerate, that we not have pain, misery, suffering- bodily, mentally, or spiritually.

Bodily and mental suffering we know. But what is spiritual suffering? To be in ignorance of the Spirit. It is present, always, though often unnoticed, in every limited creature, while bodily and mental pain come and go. What other motive of the word "binding" than the above can we ascribe to religion that is not either nonsensical or repelling? Obviously other motives, if any, must be subservient to the one given.

Is not the definition already given of religion consistent with the above-mentioned motive of the word "binding", the root meaning of religion? We said that religion, in part, consists in the permanent avoidance of pain, misery, suffering. Now religion can not lie merely in getting rid of something, such as pain, but it must also lie in getting hold of something else. It can not be purely negative but must be positive too. How can we permanently get away from pain without holding to its opposite –Bliss? Though Bliss is not an exact antonym of pain, it is, at any rate, a positive consciousness to which we can cling in order to get away from pain. We cannot, of course, forever hand in the air of a neutral feeling- that is neither pain nor the reverse. I repeat that religion consists not only in the avoidance of pain and suffering, but also in the attainment of Bliss, or God (that Bliss and god are synonymous, in one sense, will be explained later).

By looking, then, into the motive of the root meaning of religion (binding) we arrive at the same definition of religion we reached by the analysis of man's motive for action.

Religion is a question of fundamentals. If our fundamental motive is the seeking of Bliss or happiness, if there be not a single act we do, not a single moment we live, that is not determined ultimately by that final motive, should we not call this craving the most deep-seated one in human nature? And what can religion be if it is not somehow intertwined with the deepest-rooted craving of human nature? Religion, if it is to be anything that has life value, must base itself on a life instinct or craving. This is an a priori plea for the conception of religion set forth in this book.

If one replies there are many other human instincts (social, self-preservative, and so forth) besides a craving for happiness, and asks why we should not interpret religion in the light of those instincts, too, the answer is that those instincts are either subservient to the instinct of seeking happiness or are too indissolubly connected with the latter to affect substantially our interpretation of religion.

To revert once more to the former argument, *that which is universal and most necessary to man is religion to him.* If what is most necessary and universal is not religion to him, what then can it be? That which is most accidental and variable can not be it, of course. If we try to make money the one and only thing requiring attention in life, then money becomes religion to us – "the Dollar is our God". The predominant life motive, whatever it may be, is religion to us. Leave aside here the orthodox interpretation, for principles of action, and not intellectual profession of dogmas, not observance of ceremonies, determine, without the need of our personal advertisement, what religion we have. We need not wait for either the theologian or the minister to name our sect or religion for us – our principles and actions have a million tongues to tell it to us and to others.

The significant part of it all is that back of whatsoever thing we worship with blind exclusiveness is always one fundamental motive. That is, if we make money, business, or obtaining the necessities or luxuries of life the be-all and end-all of our existence, still back of our actions lies a deeper motive: we seek these things in order to banish pain and bring happiness. This fundamental motive is humanity's real religion; other secondary motives form pseudo-religions. Because religion is not conceived in a universal way it is relegated to the region of clouds, or thought to be a fashionable diversion for women, or for the aged and feeble.

Thus we see that Universal Religion (or religion conceived in this universal way) is practically or *pragmatically* necessary. Its necessity is not artificial or forced. Though in the heart its necessity is perceived, yet unfortunately we are not always fully alive to it. Had we been so, pain would long since have disappeared from the world. For ordinarily what a man thinks to be really necessary he will seek at all hazards. If the earning of money is thought by a man to be really necessary for the support of his family, he will not shrink from running into dangers to secure it. It is a pity we do not consider religion to be necessary in the same way. Instead, we regard it as an ornament, a decoration, and not a component part of man's life.

It is also a great pity that although the aim of every man in this world is necessarily religious, inasmuch as he is working always to remove want and attain happiness, yet owing to certain grave errors he has been misdirected and led to consider the true religion, the definition of which we have just given, as a thing of minor importance. What is the cause of this? Why do we not perceive the real necessity in place of the apparent unimportance? The answer is – *society*, and our inherent tendencies in an indirect way.

It is the company we keep that determines for us the necessity we feel for different things. Consider the influence of persons and circumstances. If you wish to orientalize an occidental, place him in the midst of the Asiatics; or if you want to Occidentalize an oriental, plant him among Europeans – and mark the results. It is obvious – inevitable. The man of the West learns to like the customs, habits, dress, modes of living and thought and manner of viewing things of the East, and the man of the East comes to like those of the West. The very standard of truth seems to them to vary.

Upon one thing, however, most people will agree, and that is that their worldly life, with its cares and pleasures, weal and woe, is worth living. But of the necessity for *the Universal Religion few or none* will ever remind us, and so we are not quite alive to it. It is a truism that man can not look beyond the circle in which he is placed. Whatever falls within his own circle he justifies, follows, imitates, emulates, and feels to be the standard of thought and conduct. What is beyond his own sphere he overlooks or lessens the importance of. A lawyer, for instance, will praise and be most attentive to what concerns law. Other things will, as a rule, have less importance for him.

The pragmatical or practical necessity of the Universal Religion is surely the permanent avoidance of pain and the conscious realization of Bliss, *but few understand the importance and practical necessity that this religion carries with it.*

Now it is necessary for us to investigate the ultimate cause of pain and suffering, mental and physical, in the avoidance of which the Universal Religion partly consists.

First of all we should assert, from our common universal experience, that we are always conscious of ourselves as the active power performing all of our mental and bodily acts. Indeed many different functions are we performing – perceiving, thinking, remembering, feeling, acting, and so forth. Yet underlying these functions we can perceive that there is an "ego" or "self", which governs them and thinks of itself as substantially the same through all its past and present existence. The Bible says, "Know ye not that ye are the temple of God, and that the Spirit of God dwelleth in you?" All of us as individuals are so many reflected spiritual selves of the universal *Blissful Spirit – God*, Just as there appear many images of the one sun, when reflected in a number of vessels full of water, so are we apparently divided into many souls, occupying these bodily and mental vehicles, and thus outwardly separated from the One Universal Spirit. In reality, God and man are one, and the separation is only apparent.

Now, being blessed and reflected *Spiritual selves, why is it that we are utterly unmindful of our Blissful state and are instead subject to physical and mental pain and suffering?*
The answer is that the Spiritual self has brought on itself this present state (by whatever process it may be) by identifying itself with a transitory bodily vehicle and a restless mind. The Spiritual self being thus identified, feels itself sorry for or delighted at a corresponding unhealthy and unpleasant or healthy and pleasant state of the body and mind. Because of this identification, the Spiritual self is being continually disturbed by their transitory states. To take even the figurative sense of identification: a mother who is in deep identification with her only child suffers and feels intense pain merely by the very hearing of her child's rumored or real death, whereas she may feel no such pain if she hears of the death of a neighboring mother's child with whom she has not identified herself. Now we can imagine the consciousness when the identification is real and not figurative. Thus *the sense of identification with the transitory body and restless mind is the source or root-cause of our Spiritual self's misery.*

Understanding that identification of the Spiritual self with the body and mind is the primary cause of pain, *we should now turn to a psychological analysis of the immediate or proximate causes of pain and to the distinction between pain, pleasure, and Bliss.*

Because of this identification the Spiritual self seems to have certain tendencies, mental and physical.  Desire for the fulfillment of these tendencies creates want produces pain.  Now these tendencies or inclinations are either natural or created, natural tendencies producing created wants. *A created want becomes a natural want in time, through habit.  Of whatever sort the want may be, it gives pain.*  The more wants we have, the greater the possibilities of pain.  For the more wants we have, the more difficult is it to fulfill them, and the more that wants remain unfulfilled, the greater is the pain.  Increase desires and wants, and pain is also increased.  Thus if desire finds no prospect of immediate fulfillment, or finds an obstruction, pain immediately arises.  And what is desire?  It is nothing but a new condition of "excitation" which the mind puts on itself- a whim of the mind created through company.  *Thus desire, or the increase of conditions of "excitation" of the mind, is the source of pain or misery, and also of the mistake of seeking to fulfill wants by first creating and increasing them, and then by trying to satisfy them with objects instead of lessening them from the beginning.*

It might appear that pain is sometimes produced without the presence of previous desire, for example, pain from a wound.  But we should observe here that the desire to remain in a state of health which, consciously or subconsciously, is present in our mind and is crystallized into our physiological organism, is contradicted in the above case by the presence of the unhealthy state, viz., the presence of the wound.  Thus when a certain exciting condition of the mind in the form of a desire is not satisfied or removed, pain results.

As desire leads to pain, so it leads also to pleasure, the only difference being that in the first case want involved in desire is not satisfied, while in the second case want involved in desire seems to be satisfied by the presence of external objects.  But this pleasurable experience, resulting from the fulfillment of the want by objects, does not remain but dies away, and we retain only the memory of the objects that seemed to have removed the want. Hence, in future, desire for those objects brought in by memory revives, and there arises a feeling of want which, if unfulfilled, again leads to pain.

*Pleasure is a double consciousness* – made up of an "excitation" consciousness of possession of the thing desired and of the consciousness that pain for want of the thing is felt no more. That is, there is an element of both feeling and thought in it. This latter *contrast consciousness*, i.e., the entire consciousness (how I felt pain when I did not have the desired object, and how I now have no pain, as I have obtained the thing I wanted), is what mainly constitutes for men the charm of pleasure. Hence we see that consciousness of want precedes-and consciousness of the want being fulfilled enters into-pleasurable consciousness. Thus it is want and the fulfillment of want with which the pleasure consciousness is concerned. It is mind that creates want and fulfills it.

It is a great mistake to regard a certain object as pleasurable in itself and to store the idea of it in the mind in the hope of fulfilling a want by its actual presence in the future. If objects were pleasurable in themselves, then the same dress or food would always please every one, which is not the case. What is called *pleasure* is a creation of the mind- *it is a deluding "excitation" consciousness, depending upon the satisfaction of the preceding state of desire and upon present contrast consciousness.* The more a thing is thought to excite pleasurable consciousness, and the more the desire for it is harbored in the mind, the greater the possibility of hankering after the thing itself, the presence of which is thought to bring a pleasurable consciousness and its absence a sense of want. Both of these states of consciousness lead ultimately to pain. So if we are really to lessen pain, we are, as far as possible, to free the mind gradually from all desire and sense of want. If desire for a particular thing supposed to remove the want, is banished, deluding "excitation" consciousness of pleasure does not arise, even if the thing is somehow present before us.

But instead of lessening or decreasing the sense of want, we habitually increase it and create new and various wants for the satisfying of one, resulting in a desire to fulfill them all. For instance, to avoid the want of money we start a business. In order to carry on the business we have to pay attention to thousands of wants and necessities that the carrying on of a business entails. Each want and necessity in turn involves other wants and more attention, and so on. Thus we see that the original pain involved in want of money is a thousand times multiplied by the creation of other wants and interests. Of course it is not meant that the running of a business or earning of money is bad or unnecessary. The point is that the desire to create greater and greater wants is bad.

If, in undertaking to earn money for some end we make money our end, our madness begins. For the means becomes the end and the real end is lost sight of. And so again our misery commences. In this world every one has his duties to perform. Let us, for the sake of convenience, review the former instance. The family man has to earn money to support his family, which means the doing away of his wants and those of his family. To earn money, let us suppose he starts a business and begins to attend to the details that will make it successful. Now what often happens after a time? The business goes on successfully and money perhaps accumulates until there is much more than is necessary for the fulfillment of his wants and those of his family.

Now one of two things happens. Either money comes to be earned for its own sake and a peculiar pleasure comes to be felt in hoarding, or it may happen that the hobby of running this business for its own sake persists or increases the more. We see that in either case the means of quelling original wants-which was the end- has become an end in itself-money or business has become the end. Or it may happen that new and unnecessary wants are created and an effort is made to meet them with things. In any case our sole attention drifts away from Bliss (which we, by nature, mistake for pleasure and the latter becomes our end). Then the purpose for which we apparently started business becomes secondary to the creation or increase of conditions or means. And at the root of creation or increase of conditions or means there is a desire for them which is an excitation or feeling, and also a mental picture of the past when these conditions gave rise to pleasure.

Naturally the desire seeks fulfillment by the presence of these conditions; when it is fulfilled, pleasure arises; when not fulfilled, pain arises. And because pleasure, as we remarked already, is born of desire and is connected with transitory things, it leads to excitation and pain when there is a disappearance of those things. That is how our misery commences. To put it briefly: from the original purpose of the business, which was the removal of physical wants, we turn to the means – either to the business itself or to the hoarding of wealth coming out of it – or sometimes to the creation of new wants, and because we find pleasure in these we are drawn away to pain, which, as we pointed out, is always an indirect outcome of pleasure.

What is true of the earning of money is also true of every action of the world. *Whenever we forget our true end – the attainment of Bliss or the state, condition or mode of living eventually leading to it – and direct our sole attention to the things which are mistakenly thought to be the means or conditions of Bliss, and turn them into ends, our wants, desires, excitations go on increasing, and we are started on the road to misery or pain.* We should never forget our goal. We should put a hedge round our wants. We should not go on increasing them more and more, for that will bring misery in the end. I do not mean, however, that we should not satisfy necessary wants, arising out of our relation to the whole world, or become idle dreamers and idealists, ignoring our own essential part in promoting human progress.

To sum up: pain results from desire, and in an indirect way also from pleasure, which stands as a will-o'-the-wisp to lure people away into the mire of wants to make them ever miserable.

Thus we see that desire is the root of all misery, which arises out of the sense of identification of the "self" with mind and body. *So what we should do is to kill attachment by doing away with the sense of identification.* We should break the cord of attachment and identification only. We should play our parts, as appointed by the Great Stage Manager, on the stage of the world with the whole mind, intellect, and body, inwardly as unaffected or unruffled by pleasure and pain consciousness as are the players on an ordinary stage. When there is dispassion and severing of identification, Bliss-consciousness arises in us. As long as you are human you can not but have desires. Being human, how then can you realize your divinity? First have rational desires, then stimulate your desire for nobler things, all the while trying to attain Bliss-consciousness. You will feel that the cord of your individual attachment to those desires is being automatically snapped. That is to say, from that calm center of Bliss you will ultimately learn to *disown* your own petty desires and feel only those which seem to be urged in you by a great Law. So Jesus Christ said, "Not my will, but Thine, be done."

When I say that to attain *Bliss* is the universal end of religion, I do not mean by Bliss what is usually called pleasure, or that intellectual satisfaction which arises from the fulfillment of desire and want and which is mixed with an excitation, as when we say we are pleasurably excited. In Bliss there is no excitement, nor is it a contrast consciousness, i.e., "my pain or want has been removed by the presence of such and such objects." It is a consciousness of perfect tranquility – a consciousness of our calm nature unpolluted by the intruding consciousness that pain is no more. An illustration will make the point clear. I have a wound, and feel pain; when healed I feel pleasure. This pleasurable consciousness consists of an "excitation" or feeling, and a constant thought-consciousness that I am no longer feeling the pain of the wound. Now the man who has attained Bliss, even though he might receive a physical wound, will feel, when healed, that his state of tranquility had neither been disturbed, when the wound existed, nor regained when it was healed. He feels that he is passing through a pain-pleasure universe with which he really has no connection, or which can neither disturb nor heighten the tranquil or blissful state which flows on within him without ceasing. This state of Bliss is free from both inclinations and excitement involved in pleasure or pain.

There is a positive and a negative aspect in Bliss-consciousness. The negative aspect is the absence of pleasure-pain consciousness; the positive one is the transcendental state of a superior calm, including within itself the consciousness of a great expansion and that of "all in One and One in all". It has its degrees. An earnest truth-seeker gets a little taste of it, a seer or a prophet is filled with it.

Pleasure and pain having their origin in desire and want, it should be our duty-if we wish to attain Bliss-to banish all desire except the desire for Bliss- our real nature. If all our improvements – scientific, social, and political – are guided by this one common universal end- removal of pain – why should we bring in a foreign something-pleasure- and forget to be durably fixed in what is tranquility or Bliss? He who enjoys the pleasure of health will inevitably sometimes feel the pain due to ill-health, because pleasure depends upon a condition of the mind, viz., the idea of health. To have good health is not bad nor is it wrong to seek it. But to have attachment to it, to be pleasurably or painfully affected by it, is what is objected to. For to be so means entertaining desire, which will lead to misery.

We must seek health not for the pleasure in it but because it makes the performance of duties and the attainment of our goal possible. It will, some time or other, be contradicted by the opposing condition, viz., ill-health. But Bliss depends upon no particular condition external or internal. *It is a native state of the Spirit.* Therefore it has no fear of being contradicted by any other condition. It will flow on continually forever, in defeat or success, in health or disease, in opulence or poverty.

Now the above psychological discussion about pain, pleasure, and Bliss, with the help of the following two examples, will make clear my conception of the highest common necessity and of the God-head, which was touched upon incidentally at the beginning. I remarked at the outset that if we mad a close observation of the actions of men, we should see that the one fundamental and universal motive for which man acts is the avoidance of pain and the consequent attainment of Bliss, or God. The first part of the motive, i.e., the avoidance of pain, is something we cannot deny, if we observe the motives of all the good and bad actions performed in the world.

Take the case of a person who wishes to commit suicide and that of a truly religious man who has dispassion for the things of the world. There can be no doubt about the fact that both of these men are trying to get rid of the pain which is troubling them. Both are trying to put an end to pain permanently. Whether they are successful or not is a different question, but so far as their motives are concerned there is unity.

But are all actions in this world *directly* prompted by the desire for the attainment of permanent Bliss, or God, the second part of the common motive for all actions? Does the debauchee have for his immediate motive the attainment of Bliss? Hardly. The reason for this was pointed out in the discussion about pleasure and Bliss. We found that because of the identification of the Spiritual self with the body it has fallen into the habit of indulging in desires and the consequent creation of wants. These desires and wants lead to pain, if not fulfilled – and to pleasure, if fulfilled – by objects. But here occurs a fatal error on the part of man. When a want is fulfilled, man gets a pleasurable excitement and, through a sad mistake, fixes his eye solely upon the objects which create this excitement, and supposes them to be the main causes of his pleasure. He entirely forgets that he had formerly an excitation in the form of desire or want in his won mind, and that later he had another excitation in his mind superseding the first one, in the form of pleasure which the coming of objects seems to produce. So, as a matter of fact, one excitation arose in the mind and was superseded by another in the same mind.

Outward objects are only the occasions – they are not causes. A poor person's desire for delicacies can be satisfied by an ordinary sweetmeat, and this fulfillment will give rise to pleasure. But the desire for delicacies on the part of a rich person can perhaps be satisfied only by the best of pastries, and the fulfillment will also give the *same amount of pleasure. Then does pleasure depend on outward objects, or on the state of mind? Surely the latter.* But pleasure, as we said, is an excitation. Therefore it is never justifiable to drive away the excitation in desire by another excitation, viz., that felt in pleasure. Because we do this our excitations never end, and so our pain and misery never cease.

What we should do is to set at rest the excitation that is in desire and not to fan or continue it by excitation in pleasure. This setting at rest is rendered possible, in an effective way, only by Bliss-consciousness which is not callousness but a superior stage of indifference to both pain and pleasure. *Every human being is seeking to attain Bliss by fulfilling desire, but he mistakenly stops at pleasure, and so his desires never end, and he is swept away into the whirlpool of pain.*

Pleasure is a dangerous will-o'-the-wisp. And yet it is this pleasurable association that becomes our motive for future actions. This has proved to be as deceptive as the mirage in a desert. Since pleasure, as was said before, consists of an excitation-consciousness plus a contrast-consciousness that the pain is now no more, we prepare ourselves, when we aim at it instead of at Bliss, for running headlong into that cycle of empirical existence which brings pleasure and pain in never-ending succession. We fall into terrible distress because of the change in our angle of vision from Bliss to pleasure, which latter crops up in place of the former. Thus we see that though the true aim of mankind is the avoidance of pain and the attainment of Bliss, yet owing to a fatal error man, though trying to avoid pain, *pursues a deluding something named pleasure, mistaking it for Bliss.* That the attainment of Bliss and not pleasure is the universal and highest necessity is indirectly proved by the fact that man is never satisfied with one object of pleasure. He always flies from one to another. From money to dress, from dress to property, thence to conjugal pleasure – there is a restless continuity. And so he is constantly falling into pain, even if he wishes to avoid it, by the adoption of what he deems proper means. Yet an unknown and unsatisfied craving seems ever to remain in his heart.

But a religious man (the second example which I proposed to show) always wishes to adopt proper religious means by which he can come in contact with Bliss, or God.

Of course when I say that God is Bliss, I mean also that He is ever-existent and that He is also *conscious* of His blissful existence. And when we wish Eternal Bliss or God, it is implied that with Bliss we also wish eternal, immortal, unchangeable, ever-conscious existence. That all of us, from the highest to the lowest, desire to be in Bliss has been proved *a priori*, and by a consideration of the motives and acts of men.

To repeat the argument in a slightly different way: suppose some Higher Being should come to us and say to all people of the earth, "You creatures of the world! I will give you eternal sorrows and misery along with eternal existence; will you take that?" Would any one like the prospect? Not one. All want eternal Bliss (*Anandam*) along with eternal existence (*Sat*). As a matter of fact, consideration of the motives of the world also shows there is no one but would like to have Bliss or *Anandam*. Similarly, no one likes the prospect of annihilation; if it is suggested, we shudder at the idea. All desire to exist permanently (Sat). But if we were given eternal existence without the consciousness of the existence, we would reject that. For who is there that would embrace existence in sleep? None. We all want conscious existence. Furthermore, we want *blissful conscious existence – Satchidanandam-* that is the Hindu name of God. But for a pragmatical consideration only, we emphasize the Blissful aspect of God and our motive for Bliss, leaving out two other aspects – *Sat* and *Chit, i.e., conscious existence*. Also other aspects of Him are not dwelt on here.

Now, what is God? If God be something other than Bliss, and His contact produces in us no Bliss, or produces in us only pain, or if His contact does not drive pain away from us, should we want Him? No. If God is something useless to us, we want Him not. What is the use of a God who remains always unknown and whose presence is not *inwardly* manifest to us at least in some circumstance in our life? Whatever conception of god we form by the exercise of reason or intellect, Transcendent, Immanent, et cetera, will always remain vague and indistinct unless really felt as such. In fact, we keep God at a safe distance, conceiving Him sometimes as a mere personal Being, and then again *theoretically* thinking Him to be within us. It is because of this vagueness in our idea and experience concerning God that we are not able to grasp the real necessity of God and the pragmatical value of religion. This colorless theory or idea does not bring conviction to us. It can not change our lives, influence our conduct in an appreciable way, or *make us try to know God.*

What does Universal Religion say about God? It says that the *proof of the existence of God lies in ourselves.* It is an inner experience. You can surely recall at least one moment in your life when, in prayer or worship you felt that the trammels of your body had nearly vanished, that the duality of experience – pleasure and pain, petty love and hate, et cetera – had receded from your mind. Pure Bliss and tranquility had been welling up in your heart and you were enjoying an unruffled calm – Bliss and contentment. Though this kind of higher experience does not often some to all, yet there can be no doubt of the fact that all men, at some time or other, in prayer or in mood of worship or meditation, perceive it in a less marked degree, at least.

Is this not a proof of the existence of God? *What other direct proof than the existence of Bliss in ourselves in real prayer or worship can we give of the existence and nature of God?* Though there is the cosmological proof of the existence of God- from effect we rise to cause, from the world to the World-Maker. And there is the teleological proof as well- from the telos (plan, adaptation) in the world, we rise to the Supreme Intelligence that makes the plan and adaptation. There is also the moral proof- from conscience and the sense of perfection we rise to the Perfect Being to whom our responsibility is due. Still, we should admit that these proofs are more or less the products of inference. We can not have full or direct knowledge of God through the limited powers of the intellect. Intellect gives only a partial and indirect view of things. To view a thing intellectually is not to see it by being one with it: it is to view it by being apart from it. But intuition, which we shall later explain, is the direct grasp of truth. It is in this intuition that Bliss-consciousness and God-consciousness, is realized.

*There is not a shadow of doubt as to the absolute identity of Bliss-consciousness and god-consciousness,* because when we have that Bliss-consciousness we feel that our narrow individuality has been transformed and that we have risen above the duality of petty love and hate, pleasure and pain, and have attained a level from which the painfulness and worthlessness of empirical consciousness become glaringly apparent. And we also feel and inward expansion and all-embracing sympathy for all things. The tumults of the world die away, excitements disappear, and the "all in One and One in all" consciousness seems to dawn upon us. A glorious vision of light appears. All imperfections, all angularities, sink into nothingness. We seem to be translated into another region, the fountainhead of perennial Bliss, the starting point of one unending continuity. Is not Bliss-consciousness, then, the same as God-consciousness, in which the above states of realization seem obvious?

It is evident, therefore, that God cannot be better conceived than as Bliss if we try to bring Him within the range of every one's calm experience. No longer will God be a supposition then, to be theorized over. Is this not a nobler conception of God? He is perceived as manifesting himself in our hearts in the form of Bliss in meditation – in prayerful or worshipful mood. If we conceive of God in this way, i.e., as Bliss, then and then only can we make religion universally necessary. For no one can deny that he wishes to attain Bliss and, if he wishes to achieve it in the proper way, he is going to be religious through approaching and feeling God, who is described as very close to his heart as Bliss.

This Bliss-consciousness or God-consciousness can pervade all our actions and moods, if we but let it. If we can get a firm hold on this, we shall be able to judge the relative religious worth of every minor action and motive on this earth. If we are once convinced that the attainment of this Bliss-consciousness is our religion, our goal, our ultimate end, then all doubts as to the meaning of multifarious teachings, injunctions, and prohibitions of the different faiths of the world will disappear. Everything will be interpreted in the light of the stage of growth for which it is prescribed. Truth will shine out, the mystery of existence will be solved, and a light will be thrown upon the details of our lives, with their various actions and motives. We shall be able to separate the naked truth from the outward appendages of religious doctrines and see the worthlessness of conventions that so often mislead men and create differences between them.

Furthermore, if religion is understood in this way, there is no man in the world – whether boy, youth, or an old person – who can not practice it, whatever may be the station of life to which he belongs, whether that of student, laborer, lawyer, doctor, carpenter, scholar, or philanthropist. If to abolish the sense of want and attain Bliss is religion, who is there that is not trying to be religious and will not try to be so in a greater degree, if proper methods are pointed out? Herein does not arise the question of the variety of religions – that of Christ, of Mohammed, or of the Hindus. Every one in the world is inevitably trying to be religious, and can seek to be more completely so by the adoption of proper means. There is no distinction here of caste or creed, sect or faith, dress or clime, age or sex, profession or position. For this religion is universal.

If you said that all the people of the world ought to accept the Lord Krishna as their God, would all the Christians and the Mohammedans accept that? If you asked every one to take Jesus as their Lord, would all the Hindus and Mohammedans do that? And if, again, you bade all accept Mohammed as their Lord, would all the Christians and Hindus agree to that? But if you say, "Oh, my Christian, Mohammedan and Hindu Brethren, your Lord god is Ever-Blissful Conscious Existence (Being)," will they not accept this? Can they possibly reject it? Will they not demand Him as the only One who can put an end to all their miseries?

Nor can one escape this conclusion by saying that Christians, Hindus, or Mohammedans do not conceive Jesus, Krishna, or Mohammed respectively as the Lord god – they are thought to be only the standard-bearers of God, the human incarnations of divinity. What if one thinks that way? It is not the physical body of Jesus, Krishna, or Mohammed that we are primarily interested in, nor are we so much concerned with the historical place they occupy. Nor are they memorable to us because of their different and interesting ways of preaching God. *We revere them because they knew and felt God.* It is that fact which interests us in their historical existence and in their manifold ways of expressing the truth.

They might or might not be on the same plane. Let the hard-shelled theologians and difference-hunters in religion fight over that question eternally and vainly. But did they not belong to a more or less close family of God? Did they not all realize God as Bliss and reveal real blessedness as true godliness? Is not that a sufficient bond of unity among them- let alone other aspects of Godhead and truth they might have realized and expressed? Shouldn't a Christian, a Hindu, and a Mohamedan find interest in one another's prophets, inasmuch as each of them cherished in his heart god-consciousness as primarily superior Bliss-consciousness as primarily superior Bliss-consciousness? As God unites all religions, is it not the conception and realization of Him as Bliss, if not anything else, that unites the consciousness of the prophets of all religions?

One should not think that this conception of God is too abstract, having nothing to do with our spiritual hopes and aspirations, which require the conception of God as a Personal Being. It is not the conception of an Impersonal Being, as commonly understood, nor that of a Personal Being, as narrowly conceived. God is not a Person, as are we in our narrowness. Our being, consciousness, feeling, volition have but a shadow of resemblance to His Being (Existence), Consciousness, and Bliss. He is a Person in the transcendental sense. Our being, consciousness, feeling are limited and empirical; His are unlimited and transcendental. Nor should He be thought of as Abstract, absolute, Impersonal, Unconditional, Remote, and beyond the reach of all experience- even our inner one.

*He comes within the calm experience of men. It is in Bliss- consciousness that we realize Him. There can be no other direct proof of His existence. It is in Him as Bliss that our spiritual hopes and aspirations find fulfillment – our devotion and love find an object.* No other conception of a Personal Being who is nothing but ourselves magnified is required. God may be or become anything – Personal, Impersonal, all-merciful, Omnipotent, and so forth. But we are not required to take note of these. *Whatever conception we have put forth exactly suits our purposes, our hopes, our aspirations, and our perfection.*

Nor should we think that this conception of God will make us dreamy idealists, severing our connection with the duties and responsibilities, joys and sorrows, of this practical world. If God is Bliss and if we seek Bliss to know Him, we cannot neglect the duties and responsibilities of the world. In the performance of them we can still fell Bliss, for it is beyond them, and so they cannot affect it. We transcend the joys and sorrows of the world in Bliss, but we do not transcend the duties and responsibilities in the sense of neglecting them. For in doing everything – eating, drinking, seeing, hearing, feeling, smelling, tasting, undergoing experiences, performing every minute duty of the world – we do nothing, we eat, drink, see, hear, feel, smell, taste nothing- we feel no sorrow nor pleasure. We remain unattached; all actions flow from our nature – that is human. We, bathed in an unending flow of Bliss, feel the Spiritual self to be the *dispassionate seer* of all our actions. Our narrow egoism vanishes, the All-Ego dawns, and Bliss spreads through our being. We feel that we are playing our appointed parts on the stage of the world, without being *inwardly* affected by the weal and woe, love and hate, that the playing of a part involves.

Verily, in all respects the world can be likened to a stage. The stage manager chooses people to help him in the enactment of a certain play. He allots particular parts to particular persons-all of them work according to his directions. One the stage manager makes a king, one a minister, one a servant, another the hero, and so on. One has to play a sorrowful part, another a joyful one. If each one plays his part according to the directions of the stage manager, then the play, with all its diversities of comical, serious, sorrowful parts, becomes successful. Even the insignificant parts have their indispensable places in the play.

The success of the play lies in the perfect playing out of each part. Each actor plays his part of sorrow or pleasure realistically, and to all outward appearances seems to be affected by it; but inwardly he remains untouched by it or by the passions he portrays – love, hate, desire, malice, pride, humility. But if any actor, in the playing of a part, identified himself with a certain situation or a particular feeling expressed in the play and lost his own individuality, he would be thought foolish, to say the least. A story will bring out the latter point clearly.

Once in the house of a rich man the play of *Ramayan* was staged. In the course of the play it was found that the man who should play the part of *Hanuman* (a monkey), the attendant-friend of Ram, was missing. In his perplexity the stage manager seized upon an ugly simpleton, Nilkamal by name, and sought to make him enact the part of *Hanuman*. Nilkamal at first refused, but was forced to appear on the stage. His ugly appearance excited loud laughter among the spectators and they began to shout in merriment, "*Hanuman, Hanuman!*"

Nilkamal could hardly bear this. He forgot that it was a play, and bawled out in real exasperation, "Why, Sirs, do you call me Hanuman? Why do you laugh? I am not a Hanuman. The stage manager made me come out here this way."

Nilkamal failed to distinguish between the real *Hanuman* monkey and the *Hanuman* of the play. In this world our lives are nothing but plays. But alas! We identify ourselves with the play, and hence feel disgust, sorrow and pleasure. We forget the direction and injunction of Great Stage Manager. In the act of living our lives- playing our parts – we feel as real all our sorrows and pleasures, loves and hates-in a word, we become attached, affected. This play of the world is without beginning and end. Every one must play his part, as assigned by the Great Stage Manager, ungrudgingly; must play for the sake of the play only; must act sorrowful when playing sorrowful parts, or pleased when playing pleasurable parts, but should never be *inwardly identified with the play* – with its sorrows and pleasures, loves and hates. Nor should one wish to play another's part. If every one aspires to play the role of a king, the play will be impossible.

He who has attained to the *superior* state of Bliss-consciousness will *feel* the world to be a stage and play out his part as best he can, feeling it as such, remembering the Great Stage Manager, God, and knowing and feeling His nature in its every aspect – His plan and direction.

CHAPTER III
FOUR FUNDAMENTAL RELIGIOUS METHODS

We have seen in the last chapter that the identification of the Spiritual self with body and mind is the fundamental cause of our pain, suffering, and limitations, and that because of this identification we feel such excitations as pain and pleasure, and are almost blind to the state of Bliss, or God-consciousness. We have also seen that religion essentially consists in the permanent avoidance of such pain and in the attainment of pure Bliss, or God.

As the sun's true image cannot be perceived in the surface of moving water, so the true blissful nature of the Spiritual self – the reflection of the Universal Spirit – cannot be understood owing to the waves of disquietude that arise from identification of the self with the changing states of the body and mind. As the moving waters distort the true image of the sun, so does the disturbed state of the mind, through identification, distort the true, Ever-Blissful nature of the Inner Self.

The purpose of this chapter is to discuss the easiest, most rational, and most fundamental methods, practical for all, that will free the Ever-Blissful, Spiritual self from its baneful connection and identification with the transitory body and mind, thus causing it permanently to avoid pain and attain Bliss, which constitutes religion. Therefore, the fundamental methods to be considered are religious and involve religious actions, because only by means of these can the Spiritual self be freed from the body and mind and thus from pain, and be made to attain permanent Bliss or God.

A general idea of the religious method is given in one, among a great many, of Christ's teachings. He says, "Unless ye have lifted up the Son of man, ye cannot enter into the kingdom of God." The "Son of man" means the progeny of man, i.e., *the body* which is born out of another human body. It may seem to us that "Son of man" means something other than this – that it means Christ. Granting this, we are then to interpret the next saying of Christ, "The Son of man shall be delivered unto the Gentiles and He shall be crucified," as meaning that Christ, the Eternal Spirit was to be crucified by material nails and His Spirit destroyed, an explanation which is obviously absurd; for it was the material body only, in which the Spirit of Christ was clothed, that could possibly be crucified, not the Spirit. We can explain the first quoted saying of Christ in this way: unless we can *transcend* the body and realize ourselves as spirit, we cannot enter into the kingdom or state of that Universal Spirit. We find an echo of this in a Sanskrit couplet of the Oriental scriptures: "If thou canst transcend the body and perceive thyself as spirit, thou shalt be eternally blissful and free from all pain." (When Christ called himself Son of God, he meant the Universal Spirit dwelling in him.)

Now there are *four* fundamental, universal religious methods which, if followed in daily life, will in time liberate the Spiritual self from the trammels of its bodily and mental vehicles. *Under these four* classes of religious methods I include all the possible religious practices that have ever been enjoined by any saint or savant or any prophet of God. Religious practices are inculcated by prophets in the form of doctrines. Men of limited intellect, failing to interpret the true import of these doctrines, accept their exoteric or outer meaning and gradually fall into forms, conventions, and rigid practices. This is the origin of sectarianism. Rest from work on the sabbath day was interpreted to mean complete rest from all work – even religious work. This is the danger to men of limited understanding. We should remember that we are not made for the sabbath, but that the sabbath is made for us; we are not made for rules, rules are made for us-they change as we change. We are to hold to the essence of a rule, not dogmatically to its form. Change of forms and customs constitutes for many a change from one religion to another. But the deepest import of all the doctrines of all the different prophets is often the same. Most men do not understand this.

But there is equal danger in the case of the intellectually great. They try to know the Highest Truth by the exercise of the intellect alone. But the Highest Truth can be known only by realization. Realization is something other than mere understanding. We could not possibly intellectually understand the sweetness of sugar if we had not tasted it. Just so, religious knowledge is drawn from the deepest experience of one's own soul. This we often forget when we seek to learn about God, religious dogmas, and morality. We do not seek to know these through inner religious experience. It is a pity that men of great intellectual power, successful in their use of reason in the way of discovering the deep truths of the natural sciences, and other fields of knowledge, think that they will also be able to grasp intellectually the highest religious and moral truths. It is also a pity that the intellect or reason of these men, instead of being a help, is often found to be a bar to their comprehension of the Highest Truth by the only means possible – living it in one's life.

Let us consider the four methods characterizing religious growth.

**I. Intellectual Method.** The commonly adopted, natural method, not so effective in realizing the end.

Intellectual development and progression has been natural and hence common to all rational beings. It is our self-conscious understanding which differentiates us from the lower animals, that are conscious but not self conscious. In the grades and processes of evolution we see that this consciousness gradually becomes self-consciousness – from animal consciousness self-consciousness arises. The consciousness gradually tries to free itself and tries to know itself by itself, and it is thus changed into self-consciousness. This change is due to an evolutional necessity, and the universal urge toward intellectual pursuits is due to this evolutional tendency. The Spiritual self, identified with various degrees and sorts of bodily and mental state, tries gradually and naturally to return to itself through itself.

The development of the conscious thought process is one of the methods which the Spiritual self adopts to rise above the trammels of body and mind. The effort of the Spiritual self to return to itself – its lost condition – through the development of thought-process is natural. This is the process of the world. The Universal Spirit expresses itself in different grades of development, from lower to higher. In stone and earth there is no life or consciousness as we can conceive it. In trees there is vegetative growth, an approach to life, yet no full-grown life and no conscious thought-process at all. In animals there is life and also consciousness of life. In man – the culmination point –there is life, consciousness of it, and also consciousness of the Self (i.e., Self-consciousness).

Hence it is natural for a man to develop himself through thinking reasoning, by deep study of books, by original research work, and by laborious investigations into causes and effects in the natural world. The more deeply a man engages in thought-processes, the more he can be said to be utilizing the *method* by which he has come to be what he is in the course of the world-evolution process (i.e., the method by which consciousness develops into Self-consciousness) and the nearer, knowingly or unknowingly, he approaches the Self. *For in thought we rise above the body. The deliberate following of this method will bring about sure results.* Exercise of thought in study, solely for the acquirement of knowledge of a certain thing, though to some extent improving the Self-consciousness, is not so effective as that thought-process which *has as its sole object the transcending of the body and seeing the truth.*

*One of the defects of this method* is that it is a very slow process for the Spiritual self to thus realize itself. It may involve a good deal of time. While the Spiritual self begins to apprehend Self-consciousness by this method, still it is always engaged with a series of passing mental thoughts with which it *has no relation.* Tranquillity of the spirit is something beyond thought or bodily sensation, though when once attained it overflows both.

**II. Devotional Method**. This consists in the attempt to fix the attention of the Spiritual self on one object of thought, rather than on different series of thoughts and on different subjects, as in the intellectual method. Under this method are included all forms of worship (such as prayer, *from which we must eliminate all thoughts of worldly things*), or objects of reverence. The Spiritual self must fix its attention deeply on whatsoever it chooses to concentrate on. It may be any thing that it likes. The Spiritual self may create a Personal God, an Impersonal Omnipresent god, or anything else. It must simply concentrate on one subject of thought in *good earnest.*

By this process the Spiritual self becomes gradually freed from the disturbances of vagrant thoughts – the second series of disturbances – and gets time and opportunity to think itself in itself. When we *pray* earnestly, we forget all bodily sensations and drive away all intruding thoughts that try to engage our attention.

The deeper our prayer, the more intense is the satisfaction felt, and this becomes the criterion by which we measure how far we have approached Bliss-God. As the bodily sensations are left behind and the vagrant thoughts are checked, the superiority of this over the foregoing method becomes manifest.

However, this method presents certain defects and difficulties. Owing to the long continued attachment and slavery of the Spiritual self to the body – to this deep-rooted bad habit-it ineffectually tries to turn its attention away from the sphere of bodily and mental sensations. However much one may wish to pray or engage in any form of worship with one's whole heart, one's attention is mercilessly invaded by the raiding bodily sensations and vagrant thoughts brought in by memory. In prayer we are often wholly engrossed in the consideration of the circumstances favorable to it, or we are too ready to remove any of our disturbing bodily discomforts. In spite of all our conscious efforts our bad habit, which has become a second nature to us, lords it over the Self's wishes. In spite of our wishes, the mind becomes restless, and, to paraphrase, "Wherever your mind shall be there shall be your heart be also." We are told to pray to God with all our hearts. Instead, we generally pray to God with our minds and hearts occupied with bodily and mental disturbances. Let us look for a more effective way by which our Self's effort may be made easier and be more greatly helped.

**III. Meditation Method.** This and the next method are purely scientific, involving a practical course of training, and are prescribed by great sages who have realized the truth personally in their own lives. I myself learned from one of these. There is nothing of mystery in these methods, nor anything to be dreaded as harmful. They are easy, if one is properly acquainted with them.

They will be found to be universally true. Practically –felt knowledge is the best proof of their validity and pragmatic utility.

By undergoing regularly the process of meditation till they become a habit, we can bring upon ourselves regularly the processes of meditation till they become a habit, we can bring upon ourselves a state of *conscious sleep*. We generally experience this calm and pleasurable tranquil state just when we are falling into deep sleep and approaching unconsciousness, or rising from it and approaching consciousness. In this state of conscious sleep we become free from all thoughts and outer bodily sensations, and the Self gets opportunity to think of itself – it comes into the blissful state from time to time, according to the depth and frequency of its practice of meditation. In this state we are utterly forgetful of and free from all bodily and mental disturbances which divert the Self's attention. By this process of meditation the outer organs are controlled by the controlling of the voluntary nerves, as in sleep.

But this process of meditation also has its drawbacks and defects. By this process, just as in sleep, we learn to control only our outer organs, the only difference being that in sleep the outer organs are automatically controlled, while in meditation, on the contrary, the outer organs are voluntarily controlled. This produces a state of "conscious sleep". The Spiritual self then experiences this stat of conscious sleep, being continually disturbed by the involuntary and internal organs, e.g., lungs, heart, and other organs which we mistakenly supposed to be beyond control.

We must look for a better method than this, for as long as the spiritual self can not at will shut out all *bodily sensations, even interior ones, which are the occasions of the rise of thought,* but remains vulnerable to these disturbances, it can have no hope of control nor of time or opportunity to know itself.

**IV. Organic, Scientific Method**. St.Paul said: *"I die daily"* (1 cor. 15:31). By this he meant that he knew the process of controlling the internal organs and could voluntarily free his

Spiritual self from the body and mind – an experience which ordinary untrained people only feel at final death, when the Spiritual self is freed from the worn-out body. Now by undergoing a practical and regular course of training in this scientific method the Self can be felt as being separate from the body, *without final death.*

I will give only a general idea of the process and the true scientific theory on which it is based. I set it down here from my own experience. I can say it will be found to be universally true. And I *can also safely say that Bliss, which is, as I pointed out, our ultimate end, is felt in an intense degree in the act of practicing this method. The practice of it is itself intensely Blissful – far more purely Blissful,* I venture to say, *than the greatest enjoyment that any of our five senses or the mind can ever afford us.* I do not wish to give any one any other proof of its truth than is afforded by his own experience. The more one practices it with patience and regularity, the more one feels intensely and *durably fixed in Bliss.* Owing to the persistence of bad habits, the consciousness of bodily existence, with all its memories, revives occasionally and fights against that tranquillity. If any one practices regularly and for extended periods, it can be guaranteed that in time he will find himself in a highly super-mental *state of Bliss.* We should not, however, *over-wisely* seek to *imagine* beforehand the possible results to which the process may lead, and then cease practicing the method after a short trial.

In order to make real progress the following things are necessary: First, loving attention to the subject to be learned; second, desire to learn and an earnest spirit of inquiry; third, steadfastness until the desired end is attained. If we go only half-way and then, after a short practice, reject it, the desired result will not follow. If novices in spiritual practices try to prejudge the experience of experts, they will appear as ridiculous as a child who tries to imagine what post-graduate studies would be like.

It is a great pity that men will spend their best efforts and time in securing what is needed for worldly existence or in indulging in intellectual controversy over theories, but seem never to think it worth their while to realize and patiently experience in life the truths which not only vivify but impart meaning to it. Misguided efforts can engage their attention longer than well-guided efforts. I have been practicing the above-mentioned method for many years, and the more I do so, the more I feel the joy of a state of permanent and unfailing Bliss. We should bear in mind that the Spiritual self has been in bondage to the body for how many ages we know not. It cannot be freed in one day, nor will short or desultory practice of the method take one to the Supreme state of Bliss or give one control over the internal organs. It will require *patient* practice for a *long, long time.* This can be guaranteed, however – that the following of this process will bring the great joy of pure Bliss-consciousness. The more we practice it, the more we get that Blissful state. I wish that, as seekers of Bliss, which all of us are, you should try to experience for yourselves that universal truth which is in all and may be felt by all. This is not an invention of anyone. It is already there. We are simply to discover it.

Do not, until you have tested this truth, look upon what I write with indifference. It may be that you are tired of hearing various theories, none of which has hitherto had any direct bearing on your life. This is no theory, but realized truth. I am trying to give you a general idea of what can be really experienced.

I had the fortune to learn this "holy, scientific truth" from a great saint of India many years ago. You may ask why I urge you – why I draw your attention to these facts. Have I any selfish interest? To this I answer in the affirmative. I wish to give this truth to you with the hope of getting in return pure joy by helping you to find your joy in the practice and realization of it.

Now I have to enter into a little physiology, which will enable us to understand the method, at least in a general way. I must describe the work of the main centers and the electrical current that flows from the brain through these centers to the outer and internal organs and keeps them vibrating with life.

There are six main centers through which Pranic Current, Vital Current, or Life Electricity from the brain is discharged throughout the nervous system. These are:

Medulla center          Lumbar center
Cervical center         Sacral center
Dorsal center           Coccygeal center

The brain is the supreme electrical Power House (supreme center). All the centers are connected with one another and act under the influence of the supreme center (brain cells). The brain cells discharge life current, or electricity, through these cells, which in turn discharge electricity to the different efferent and afferent nerves which respectively carry motor impulses and sensations of touch, sight, and so forth. *This electrical flow from the brain is the life of the organism (of its internal and external organs), and it is this electrical medium through which all our sensation reports reach the brain and cause thought disturbances.*

The Self, if it wishes effectively to shut out the disturbing reports reports of bodily sensations (which are also the occasions of the rise of the thought-series), must control and concentrate the electrical flow and draw it back from the nervous system as a whole to the seven main centers (including the brain), so that by this process it may give the outer and internal organs perfect rest. In sleep, the electrical conductivity between the brain and the outer organs is partially inhibited, so that ordinary sensations of sound, touch, and so forth, cannot reach the brain. But because this inhibition is not complete, a sufficiently strong stimulus from without restores this electrical conductivity and is reported to the brain, awakening the person. Yet always in sleep there is a steady electrical flow into the internal organs-heart, lungs, et cetera – so that they keep on throbbing and working.

As the control of life electricity in sleep is not complete, bodily sensations of discomfort, disease, or strong outside stimuli disturb it. But through a scientific process of control, which cannot be here described in detail, we can simultaneously control the external and internal organs of the system in a perfect way. That is the ultimate result of practice. But it may take long years to attain that perfect control. As after sleep, which is rest, the outer organs are invigorated, so the internal organs, after rest, as a result of the practice of this scientific method, are greatly vitalized, and with the consequent increase in their working power, life is prolonged. As we do not fear to go to sleep, lest for the time being the outer organs remain inert, so we ought not to fear to practice conscious death, i.e., give rest to the internal organs. Death will then be under our control; for when we think this bodily house is unfit and broken, we shall be able to leave it of our own accord. "The last enemy that shall be destroyed is death." (1 Cor. 15:26)

We may describe the process thus: If the main telephone office in a town is permanently connected by wires with different parts of the town, men telephoning from those parts can always, even against the will of the authorities of the main telephone office, send messages to the central office through the medium of the electric current running along the connecting wires. If the main telephone office wishes to stop communication with the different parts, it can turn off the main electrical switch and there will be no flow to the different quarters of the town. Similarly, the scientific method teaches a process enabling us to draw to its distributed through out the organs and other parts of the body.

The process, roughly speaking, lies in magnetizing the spinal column, which contains the seven main centers, with the result that the distributed life electricity is drawn back to the original centers of discharge and is experienced in the form of light. In this state the Spiritual self can consciously free itself from its bodily and mental disturbances. The Spiritual self is, as it were, being disturbed, even against its wish, by the telephone reports from two classes of people-gentlemen (thoughts) and low class people – (bodily sensations). In order to break connection with them it has only to draw away the electricity flowing through the telephone wires to the central battery of its house by turning off the switch (i.e., practicing the fourth method), in order to enjoy relief.

*Attention is the great director and discharger of energy.* It is the active cause of the discharge of the electrical life current from the brain to the sensory and motor nerves. For example, we drive away a troublesome fly by discharging, through the power of attention, the proper electrical current along the motor nerves. For example, we drive away a troublesome fly by discharging, through the power of attention, the proper electrical current along the motor nerves, thereby producing the desired movements. I cite this to give an idea of the power by which the electrical flow of the system can be controlled and drawn back to its seven centers. It is of these seven star-like centers and their mystery that we find mention in the chapter on Revelation in the Bible. St. John experienced these seven centers as seven stars while he was in the Spirit. "The mystery of the seven stars which thou sawest, write them in an book." (Revelation 1:19, 20.) It should be noted that when I say the electrical flow of the body is controlled, I mean all electrical currents, whether flowing voluntarily or involuntarily.

In conclusion I wish to describe the nature of the states which emerge when the electrical flow is *completely* controlled. In the beginning a most attractive sensation is felt in the course of magnetizing the spinal column. But continued and long practice will bring about a state of conscious Bliss which counteracts the exciting state of our body-consciousness. *This blissful state has been described as our universal aim and highest necessity, because in it we are really conscious of God, or Bliss,* and feel the expansion of our real selves. The more frequently this is experienced, the more our narrow individuality falls away, the sooner the state of universality is reached, and the closer and more direct is our touch with what we know as God.

Religion is really nothing but the merging of our individuality in universality. Therefore, in the consciousness of this Blissful state we ascend the steps of religion. We leave the noxious atmosphere of the senses and vagrant thoughts and come to a region of heavenly Bliss. We learn by this process what will be found to be universally true. When by constant practice the consciousness of this Blissful state of the Spiritual self becomes real we find ourselves always in the holy presence of the Blissful God in us. We discharge our duties better, having an eye more for the duties themselves than for our "egoism" and the pleasure-pain-consciousness rising therefrom. Then we can solve the mystery of existence and impart real meaning to life.

Underlying the teachings of all religions – Christianity, Mohammedanism Hinduism – there is one truth remaining, viz., that unless you know yourself as spirit – as the fountain head of Bliss, separate from body and mind – your existence is devoid of meaning and your life is akin to that of the brute. We can know God only by knowing ourselves, for our natures are similar to His. Man has been created in the image of God. If the methods here suggested are learned and earnestly practiced, you will know yourself to be a Blissful spirit and will realize god. In these things there is nothing that is found in Christianity and not also in Mohammedanism and Hinduism, nothing in the latter that is not in the former.

Further, the methods laid down embrace all the conceivable means essential to the realization of God. They do leave out of consideration the thousand and one conventional rules and minor practices enjoined by the so-called different religions, because some of these relate to differences in the frame of mind of the individuals, hence are less important, though by no means unnecessary, and because others come up in the course of practice of these methods, hence do not require fuller treatment in the limited space here.

The superiority of this method over others lies in the fact that it lays its hand just on the thing that binds us down to our narrow individuality -the *life-force* that, instead of being turned back and absorbed into the expansive self-conscious force of the Self, goes outward, keeps the body and mind always in motion, and causes disturbances to the Spiritual self, in the shape of bodily sensations and passing thoughts. Because the *life-force* moves outward, sensations and thoughts disturb and distort the calm image of Self-consciousness. This method teaches us to turn the life-force inward. Hence it is direct and *immediate*. It takes us straight to the consciousness of this Self- Bliss-God. It does not require the help of an intermediary. It controls and directs the course of the life-force by the control and regulation of a known and directly connected *manifestation* of the life-force itself. (It is not desirable nor is it possible that this process be explained further in this book.)

The other methods employ the help of the intellect, or thought process, to control the *life-force* in order to induce consciousness of the Self in its Blissful and other aspects. It should be noted that all religious methods in the world directly or indirectly, tacitly or expressly, enjoin the control, regulation, and turning back of the *life-force* so that we may transcend the body and mind and know the Self in its native state. The fourth method directly controls itself by itself, whereas the other methods do it indirectly through some other intermediary – thought, prayer, good works, worship or meditation.

Presence of life in man is existence, absence of it is death. Hence the method that teaches life's direct power to control itself must be the best of all.

Now savants of different ages and climes have suggested methods adapted to the mental frame and condition of the people among whom they lived and preached. Some have laid stress on prayer, some on feeling, some on good works, some on love, some on reason or thought, some on meditation. But their motives have been the same.

They all meant that body should be transcended by the control and turning back of the *life-force* inward, and that the Self should be realized as the image of the sun in a calm, unruffled water. Their purpose is the inculcation of just that which the fourth method teaches directly, without the help of any intermediary.

At the same time it should be noted that the practice of this method does not prevent the cultivation of the intellect, the building up of the physique, and the activity of a social and useful life – a life of the best feelings and motives, devoted to philanthropic works.

As a matter of fact, *all-sided training* should be prescribed for all. It positively helps rather than retards the practice of the method; the only thing required is that its point of view be retained. Then all actions, all pursuits, will result to our advantage.

The main thing in this process, in a word, is to understand thoroughly the mystery of the life-force that sustains the bodily organism man, causing it to vibrate with life and energy, illumine the intellect, and build up a strong physique, for the creation of the ideal social man. Unless we understand what we are and what the life with which we have daily connection means, our knowledge is imperfect. So I say we should analyze the life of man, as it were, in a laboratory, find out what it is, and then devise means to make it what it ought to be. This process is not of my own invention; it has been found to be universally true in all climes and ages. Truth is always found to be the same everywhere and by every one. Only, sometimes it is out of our sight. Though seeing, we see not, hearing, we hear not. I have only wished to relate what I have found through the help of others.

CHAPTER IV
INSTRUMENTS OF KNOWLEDGE

*Perception- Inference-Intuition*

The universality and necessity of the religious ideal (ever-existent, ever-conscious Bliss-God) and the practical methods to reach it have been discussed in the previous chapters. Now we wish to discuss validity of the methods. The methods are essentially practical, and if they are followed the ideal must be reached. Whether we deal with the theories or not. Their validity is shown by the practical result itself, which is palable and real. It is not, be it understood, really necessary to show the theoretical grounds of validity. But simply to satisfy others we treat *a priori* of the validity of the theories of knowledge on which the methods are based, that their validity may also be theoretically shown.

This will launch us into the epistemological question: How and how far can we know the ideal, the truth? To show how we know the ideal we must consider how we know the actual world. We must deal with the process of knowing the world. There must deal with the process of knowing the world. There we shall see whether the process of knowing the world is the same as the process of knowing the ideal, and whether the actual world is separate from the ideal or whether the latter pervades the former, only the process of knowing the two being different. Before proceeding further let us discuss the "instruments" of knowledge – the way by which knowledge of the world is made possible to us.

There are three *instruments* or means of knowledge: *Perception, Inference, Intuition.*

**I. Perception.** Our senses are, as it were, windows, through which stimuli from the outside come and strike the mind, which passively receives these impressions. Unless the mind operates, no impression can be made on it by the stimuli coming from the outside through the sense-windows. Mind not only furnishes the connections to the stimuli received through the different senses, but stores their influences in the form of impressions. But these impressions remain a confused, disconnected mass until the discriminative faculty (*Buddhi*) operates on the impressions. A relevant connection is then established and the details of the outer world are recognized as such. They are projected, so to speak, and known in the forms of time and space, having distinct associations- quantity, quality, measure, and meaning. A house is then known as a house, and not as a post. This is the result of the operation of the Intellect (*Buddhi*).

First we see an object, feel it, and then hear the sound of it when struck, our mind receiving these impressions and storing them. *Buddhi* interprets them and seems to project them in the form of a house with its various parts – size, shape, color, form, fashion, and its relation to others in the present, past, or future – in time and space. This is how knowledge of the world arises. An insane person has impressions stored in this mind, but stored in his mind, but they are in a chaotic state – not sorted and made up into distinct, well-ordered groups by the intellect.

Now comes the question: can reality (the ideal, ever-conscious, ever-existent, Bliss-God) be known by perception of this sort? Is the process of knowing this world, viz., by perception, valid in the matter of knowing the highest truth?

Now we know the intellect can work only upon the materials supplied by the senses. It is certain that the senses give us only the stimuli of qualities and variety. Not only do the senses give variety, but intellect itself deals with variety and remains in the region of variety. Though it can think of "unity in diversity," it cannot be one with it. This is its drawback. Perception can not really give the true nature of the One, Universal Substance underlying diverse manifestations.

This is the verdict of reason itself. When *Buddhi* turns back upon itself to judge how far it is capable of knowing Reality by interpreting the sense-impressions, it finds itself hopelessly confined within the domain of the sense-world. There is no loop-hole through which it can peep into the super-sensuous world.

Some may say that because we drive a wedge worlds, reason can not bring itself to believe that it can have any knowledge of the super-sensuous. They say that if we think of the super-sensuous as manifesting in and through the sensuous, then in knowing the sensuous – with its connection (teleology, or adaptation) and all the details and varieties by the processes of the intellect – we shall be knowing the super-sensuous manifested as "unity in diversity." But it may be questioned, what is the nature of that *knowing*? Is it merely an idea in the brain, or is it *seeing* the truth (unity in diversity) face to face, first-hand and direct? Does that form of *knowing* carry the same conviction which being one with it would carry? Surely not, for that *knowing* is very partial, defective. It is merely looking through a colored glass. The super-sensuous world lies beyond. These are the *a priori* arguments against perception as an instrument for knowing Reality, or God.

From calm experience, also, we find that we can not attain that Blissful state, which is Reality and the ideal itself, as shown in the previous chapters, until we rise to a considerable extent from the restless, perceptual stage. The more we leave behind the disturbing perceptions and interior thoughts, the greater is the possibility of the dawning of that supermental state of Bliss, or Bliss-God. Ordinary perception and Bliss seem to be mutually exclusive in common experience. However, none of our methods are based on pure perception, hence the inability of the latter to know Reality does not affect the former.

**II. Inference.** This is another way of deriving knowledge of the world. But inference itself is based on experience – on perception – be it deductive or inductive. In our experience we find fire wherever there is smoke; hence if we see smoke on any occasion, we infer there is fire. This is deductive inference. But it is possible only because of our previous experience (perception) of smoke as being associated with fire. In inductive inference, also, there is the same dependence on perception.

We observe that a certain kind of bacillus is the cause of cholera. We find out the causal connection between that kind of bacillus and cholera and at once inductively infer that wherever we find this bacillus, cholera will be present. While there is a leap here from the known cases of cholera to the unknown cases, still by inference we get no new fact, though the cases may be new. The very possibility of the establishment of causal connection between bacilli and cholera depended upon observation (perception) of certain cases. So inference ultimately depends upon perception. In inferred cases we do not get any new truth – nothing really new that was not found in observed cases. In observed cases, too, bacilli are followed by cholera- no new truth, though the cases are fresh and new.

So in all forms of thought, reasoning, inference, or imagination we are not face to face with Reality. Reason or thought may arrange and systematize facts of experience. It can endeavor to see things as a whole. It may try to penetrate into the mystery of the world. But its effort is hampered by the materials on which it works – facts of experience, sense impressions. They are bald, hard facts, disconnected, limited by our powers of perception. The materials disturb rather than help the thought process, which also has a restless continuity.

The first method, as we pointed out, is the intellectual method. It busies itself with the thought process in order to know reality – the state of Bliss and calm realization. But it fails. Bodily perceptions disturb, and the thought process also, due to its working on varied, restless sense-impressions, forbids our remaining for long in a concentrated state, that we may know and feel that calm condition of Bliss and have the consciousness of unity in diversity. One merit of the Intellectual Method is that when we are absorbed in the thought-world, to a certain extent we transcend bodily sensations. But this is always temporary.

In the other two methods – Devotion and Meditation – the thought process is less. Still, it is present. In the Devotional Method, i.e., in ritual worship or otherwise, in prayer, congregational or individual, much of the thought-process is engaged in the arrangement of favorable conditions. Still there is the attempt to concentrate on some subject of worship or prayer. So far as the diversity in thought processes is checked or prevented, the devotional method is successful. Still the defect is this: due to a bad habit, confirmed in the course of ages, our concentration is not deep, leaving the possibility of setting the diversity of thought-processes at work on the slightest disturbance.

In the Meditation Method outward formalities, conventions, rites, et cetera, being dispensed with, thus barring the possibility of the thought-processes being set into motion as easily as in the Devotional Method, concentration is fixed on one object of thought. And there is a gradual tendency to leave the sphere of thought to step into that of intuition, which we shall next consider.

**III. Intuition.** So far we have been considering the instruments and processes of knowing this sensuous world. Intuition, with which we now deal, is the process by which we know the super-sensuous world – the world that is beyond senses and thoughts. It is true that the super-sensuous expresses itself in and through the sensuous, and to know the latter in completeness is to know the former, but the process of knowing the two must be different.

To know the sensuous, perception and thought will be fairly sufficient, but to know the super-sensuous, intuition is required. It is no argument to say that through the sensuous, the processes of knowing the latter (perception and thought) will also hold good in the case of the former. For, are we able to know *even the sensuous world*, in all its fullness, by these processes? Assuredly not. There is an infinite number of facts, things, laws, connections in nature, and even in our own organism, which are still – and probably ever will be – a sealed book to mankind. Far less, then, shall we be able to know what is really beyond sense-perception and thought-perception by mere sense and thought.

*Intuition comes from within; thought from without. The former gives a face-to-face view of Reality; the latter gives an indirect view of it. Intuition, by a strange sympathy, sees Reality in its totality, while thought chops it up into parts.* Every man has the power of intuition, as he has the power of thought. As thought can be cultivated, so intuition can be developed. Intuition we are in tune with Reality – with the world of Bliss, with the "unity in diversity," with the inner laws governing the spiritual world, with God.

How do we know that we exist? Through sense-perception? Do the senses first tell us that we *exist* – whence the consciousness of existence comes? That can never be. For the consciousness of existence is pre-supposed in the attempt of the senses to let us know of *our existence*. Sense cannot consciously sense anything without our first knowing that we exist in the very act of sensing. Does inference, the thought-process, tell us that *we* exist? Assuredly not. For the materials of thought must be sense-impressions, which, as we have just found, cannot tell us of our existence, as that feeling is already pre-supposed in them.

Nor can the process of thought give us the consciousness of existence, for the latter is already implied in the former. When, by comparing ourselves with the outer world, we endeavor to think or infer that *we exist* therein, the consciousness of existence is already present in the very act of thinking and inferring. Then, if sense or thought fails, how do we know that *we exist*? It is only by intuition that we can know this. This knowing is *one form* of intuition. It is beyond sense and thought – they are made possible by it.

It is very difficult to define intuition, for it is too near to every one of us. Every one of us feels it. Do we not know what the consciousness of existence is? Every one know it. It is too familiar to admit of definition. Ask one how he knows *he exists*. He will remain dumb. He knows it, but he cannot define it. He may try to explain, but his explanation does not reveal what he inwardly feels. *Intuition of every form has this peculiar character.*

The fourth method, explained in the last chapter, bases itself on intuition. The more earnest we are about it, the wider and sure will be our vision of Reality – God. It is through intuition that humanity reaches Divinity, that the sensuous is brought into connection with the super-sensuous, and that the latter is *felt* to express itself in and through the sensuous. The influence of senses vanishes, intruding thoughts disappear, Bliss-god is realized, the consciousness of "all in One and One in all" dawns upon us. This intuition is what all great savants and prophets of the world had and still have.

The third, or Meditation Method, as explained in the last chapter, also carries us into the region of intuition – when it is earnestly practiced.  But it is a bit roundabout, and ordinarily takes a longer time to produce in us the successive states of the intuitional or realization process.

Thus it is by intuition that God can be realized in *all His aspects*. We have no sense that can reveal knowledge of Him.  The senses give knowledge of only His manifestations.  No thought or inference can enable us to know Him as He truly is.  For thought cannot go beyond what the senses give.  It can only arrange and interpret the impressions of the senses.  When the senses are unable, thought, as depending  upon them, is also unable to bring us to god.  So it is to intuition that we shall have to turn for the knowledge of god in His blissful and other aspects.

Religion is truly an act of intuition ; without it the former degrades into the observance of lifeless conventions and rites.  It is from the point of view of intuition that every fact of the world finds meaning in its totality.  The

Criterion of development in the spiritual world is also intuition. Men of the world will notice whether or not you are punctual, regular, and devoted in the matter of observing the codes and canons of worldly-wise morality and religion, but the seer of truth will mark how far you have progressed in the path of realization – intuition.

However, there are many bars to this intuitional point of view – to the realization of truth.  These are some of them: disease, mental incapacity, doubt, indolence, worldly-mindedness, false ideas, and instability.

These are either inherent or engendered and aggravated through association with others.  Besides the above there may be many other inherent tendencies *(Samskaras)* which turn out to be the causes of these.  We seem to have no control over our *Samskaras*, but our strong-minded effort (*Purushakara*) can work wonders. It can change them, nay, it can destroy them. When they are changed for the better they help rather than retard us. It is through effort, as facilitated by association with the good, that new tendencies (Samskaras) can be formed and the bad ones changed.

*Until we associate with those who have seen, felt, and realized true religion in their lives we can not fully know what it is, and in what its universality and necessity lie.*

The spirit of inquiry is in all. Everyone in the world is a seeker after truth. It is his immortal heritage, and he seeks it, blindly or wisely, until he has fully reclaimed it. It is never too late to mend or seek. Search, and you will find; "Knock, and it shall be opened unto you."

# Songs of the Soul

Songs of the Soul

## CONTENTS

The Essence of Kriya Yoga

Songs of the Soul

Life's Dream
Luther Burbank


*Part IV*
Forward
Vision of Visions

The Essence of Kriya Yoga

## CONSECRATION

At Thy feet I come to shower
All my full heart's rhyming flower,
Of Thy breath born,
By Thy love grown,
With my lonely seeking found,
By hands Thou gavest picked and bound;-
For Thee the sheaves
Within these leaves:-
Of my life's season
The choicest flowers,
With petals soulful spread,
Their humble perfume shed;-
Hands folded now I come to give
What's Thine - receive!


## SOUL IS MARCHING ON

The shining stars are sunk in darkness,
The weary sun is dead at night,
The moon's soft smile doth fade anon,-
But still my soul is marching on.

The grinding wheel of Time has crushed
Full many a life of moon and star
And many a brightly smiling morn;-
But still my soul is marching on

The flowers bloomed, then hid in gloom,
The bounty of the trees did cease,

Colossal men have come and gone;-
But still my soul is marching on.

The aeons one by one are flying,-
The arrows one by one are gone,
Dimly, slowly life is fading,-
But still my soul is marching on.

Darkness, death and failures vied-
To block my path they fiercely tried;
My fight with jealous Nature's strong;-
But still my soul is marching on.


## THEY ARE THINE

I have nothing to offer Thee,
For all things are Thine;
I grieve not that I cannot give,
For nothing is mine, for nothing is mine;
Here I lay at Thy feet
My limbs, my life, my thoughts and speech,
For they are Thine, for they are thine.


## THOU IN ME

When I smile
Thou dost smile through me;
When I cry
In me Thou dost weep,
When I wake

The Essence of Kriya Yoga

Thou greetest me,
When I walk
Thou art with me.
Thou dost smile and weep,
Thou dost wake and walk
Like me; my Likeness Thou;
But when I dream,
Thou are awake;
When I stumble,
Thou art sure;
When I die
Thou art my life.


THY CALL

When lost I roam
I hear Thy call to home –
In whistling breeze
Or rustling leaves of trees.

When drunk in folly
I wander gaily
By the sandy shore, -
Who wakes me with a sudden roar?

When clouds do spread a veil
My precious joy to steal, -
Who tears the sheet away
To burst in redd'ning ray?

Songs of the Soul

When dark night blinds,
And my movements binds, -
Who shows my path and th' dark beguiles
With mildly mocking moonlit smiles?

The million starry stares,
The waking sunny glares,
The river's ever-murmuring air
Thy sure and silent call declare.


## ONE THAT'S EVERYWHERE

The tree sighs,
The wind plays,
The sun smiles,
The river moves;
Feigning dead the sky is blushing red
At the creeping sun's gentle tread.
The earth changes robes
Of black and star-lit night
For dazzling golden light.
Dame Nature loves herself t'array
In changing seasons' colors gay;
The murmuring brook e'er tries to tell
In lisping sounds so well
Of the hidden thought
By inner spirit brought.
The birds aspire to sing
Of things unknown that swell within.
But man first speaks in language true
Both loud and clear, with meaning new,

The Essence of Kriya Yoga

Of what all else before
Had failed to full declare:-
Of One That's everywhere.


WHISPERS

Leaves do sigh,
They can not speak
Of One that's high
The birds do sing,
They can not say
What in their bosom springs.
The beasts do howl
With muffled soul;
They can never say as nigh
As doth in their feelings lie.
Since I can sing or say or cry
I will mighty try
To pour out whispers Thine, - one and each
That to heart doth softly reach.


IN ME

Hello, yonder Tree!
Thou dost breathe in me, in me;
O Fast-footed River!
Thy shining meandering quiver
Declares itself
Through myself;
Thou dost shine through me, in me.

Songs of the Soul

O huge Himalaya
With snowy sovereign white regalia!
In my mind doth rest thy throne-
Thy home
In me, in me.
O Ocean! Endless to the eye
In  boundless stretches thou dost lie;
But to me thou art small;
A tiny drop upon a ball,
Thou art in me, in me.
O Endless Sky!
So vast to eye,-
In some brighter age or day
When I'll cast my cares away
On thee will sail my better boat, bright and gay,
On to thy shore
To find, I'm sure,
Thy border land – in me.
O Distant heav'ns!
O Secret One and Angels Seven!
In my sphere you all I see,
In me, in me, in me!


TOO NEAR

I stood in silence
To worship Thee
In the temple large
With blue etheric dome,
Lighted by the spangling stars,
Shining with the lustrous moon,

The Essence of Kriya Yoga

Tapestried with the golden clouds,
Where reigns no dogma loud.
I prayed and waited
For Thee to come.  I cried,-
Thou didst not come.
I will wait no more,
Nor send my feeble prayer
Footsteps Thine to hear,-
They are not heard without,
In me Thou art, - too near.

EVASION

When I do almost see Thee
Thou dost suddenly vanish;
When Thou art almost trapped in me
I find Thee gone.
When I think I have seized Thee
Thou dost most escape.
How long this hide and seek, and play?
I am weary with the toil of the day;
Still I may brook this evasion Thine
If 'tis for a tiny flash of time,
That in the end I may see
Thy face with doubled joy and mind more free.

THY CRUEL SILENCE

I prayed to Thee
But Thou wert mute,
At Thy door I knocked,

Songs of the Soul

Thou answered'st not,
I gave my tears
To soft'n Thy heart;
In cruel silence
Didst Thou watch,
But now I learn
The way to earn
Attention thine;
I'll weep and pray
Unceasingly-
In cruel silence-
Till time is old,
And earth grows cold,
Till life doth fail,
Till body fall;
Then if Thou speak'st
And dost wish me peace;-
Still I pray and weep
In cruel silence deep.


I AM HERE

I roamed alone by ocean's shore
And watched; the wrestling, brawling waves did roar
Alive with Thy own restless Life.
Thy angry mood and ripply quiver,
Thy wrathful vastness made me shiver;
I turned away from heated strife.-
A kindly waving tree
Caught my roving eye so free
To comfort me with gentler look sublime

That I did feel was Thine-
I saw the gaugeless mystic sky,
And down its valley dark I ran to pry
At Thee, and play with Thee;-
I failed to find Thy hiding Body,
Yet I felt everywhere
That Thou wert always near,
Playing at hid and seek with me,-
Receding when I almost touched Thee
As to find Thee I groped blindfold —
In ignorant darkness old.
I left my search in dim despair;
Thou royal, sly Eluder!-
In haste I hied away from Thee
And I retired within me;
When lo! Some Unseen Hand
Did quickly snatch away the all-black band
That did my eyes enfold
That were so numb and cold,
And in troth I felt quite keen;
Someone beside me stood unseen
And whispered to me, cool and clear,
"Hello, playmate, I am here1"


WHERE I AM

Not the lordly, domes on high
With tall heads daring clouds and sky,
Nor alabaster shining floors,
Nor the rich organ's awesome roar,
Nor rainbowed windows' beauty quaint

Songs of the Soul

With colossal chronicles told in paint,
Nor torch nor incense' curling soar,
Nor pure-dressed children of the choir,
Nor well-planned sermon,
Nor loud-tongued prayer
Can call Me there
The richly carven door,
Through which all pomp and pride pour,
I deign not through to go;-
But still I come Incognito.
The stony, polished altar
Or narrow builded sermon seat
Too narrow seems to hold
My large, large Body for retreat,
A humble magnet-call.
A whisper by the brook
On grassy altar small-
There I have my nook;-
A crumbling temple shrine,
A little place unseen,
Unwashed, unhedged,
Is where I humble rest and lean:
A sacred heart
Tear washed and true
Doth draw me with its rue,
I take no bribe
Of strength or wealth
Of caste or church or scribe,
Of fame or faith or festive breath,
But wail for truth;
And e'er the broken distant heart
Doth draw me e'en to heathen lands,

And My help in silence I impart.
ONE FRIEND

Many clouds do race to hide Thee-
Of friends and wealth and fame-
And yet through mist of tears I see
Appear thy Golden name.
Each time my father, mother, friends
Do loudly claim they did me tend,
I wake from sleep to sweetly hear
That Thou alone didst help me here.


## FLOWER OFFERING

A goblet of my folly-blood
Is humbly set beneath thy Petal feet,-
    O, Lotus Sweet!
I've stood with tears seeking Thine angry thirst
    to quench,-
        With sandal sweet, with motley costumed
           flowers;
        With devotion's perfume from my heart
           of hearts,
        With myrrh of constancy my soul
           imparts-
        To worship thee, Unheard is my lay,-
        And for naught I pray,-
        But with sleepless care
        I'll lay my flower there.

## THE TATTERED DRESS

I see Thy magic Hands of Death
Snatch away in stealth
And change the tattered dress,
(Which fondly men caress
With blind attachment.)
Into soul-sheen habiliment,-
This newly given robe-
That shines with all the beauties of Thy globe.

## THY SECRET THRONE

Behind the screen
Of all things seen
How dost Thou hide,-
Elude the tide
Of marching human eyes,
That 'round Thee rushing hies?
'Twill not be long
Ere will be known
Thy hiding place
By children with Thine eyes and grace.

Sage science splits
Each atom knit
By Thee, to find apace
Thy hiding place,
Is heart of atom, - electron,
Thy secret throne?

The Essence of Kriya Yoga

Deep we bore
To find Thy art, and lore
Of doings all sublime;
E'er hidden betimes.
Yet Thy abode
Seems far remote;
'Tis still to find
With deeper mind.


## METHOUGHT I HEARD A VOICE

Singing by the rill
My voice doth thrill
With echoes of my thought
By fancies brought.

I wandered in my play
On faerie fields away;
I stopped to muse, rejoice;-
Methought I heard a voice!

The flowers of that field
Of wondrous hues,- perfumed
With essence of the heart- did yield
Delicious joys undreamed.

Behind the thin bright veil
Of scented feelings
I saw some fitful flash:
Some Glistening Presence rush.

I tiptoe stood,
Listening, watching;
I poured my heart,
Listening, watching.


## A MILK-WHITE SAIL

A milk white, tiny sail
Skims fast across my sea; I wail
The threatening storms to see;-
But my bark glides free toward the lee,
So near the shore
And safe from the angry roar.


## THE HARVEST

Drawn by joy sublime
I watch each harvest time,
When the sky glows red with ripe sunbeams;
Oh, ne'er before had I found thy ploughing teams.
The oriole's painted, glowing breast is shown,
Yet thy brush, O Painter, ne'er is known
The north star timely leaps,
And its nocturnal watch unfailing keeps;
The sun and seasons Thy house supervise,
Yet thou, O Master, seemest not to rise!

## THE SPLINTERS OF THY LOVE

The splinters of Thy love
Lie strewn in many a heart:
The little fragments of Thy love,
Descended from far above,
I find spread here and there, and charm'd I start
To seize all and with care collect.
I feel as I reflect
That I have certes seen somewhere
Thy whole unbroken love that's everywhere;
And with devotion strong
I weld my varied collection
Of tiny bits of parental, friendly love in one
To match it with thy own.

## FOR THEE AND THINE

I love to seek
What's mine.
I think, I act-
I work with tact
To gain what's mine.

I pass by th' river
In joyous quiver
To soothe this mind of mine.
I smell the flowers
To cheer the hours,-

## Songs of the Soul

I love to have what's mine.
I sip the gold sunshine
To warm this flesh of mine.
I drink the fresh and flowing air,
For me I lift my prayer,
I try to rake
The world to take
All things for me and mine.-

Those dark days are gone,-
The old time's flown,
So lived for me and mine,-
In new-born light
I see what's right,-
To live for Thee and Thine.

## WAKE, WAKE, MY SLEEPING HUNGER WAKE!

When tables large of earth and moon and meteors,
Of brooks and rills, of shining ether ore
Are laid with wondrous One Nectar,
Stolen from nature's nooks by lars,-
Do thou thy sullen sleep forsake;-
Wake, wake my sleeping Hunger, wake!

Through diverse paths of aeons thou hast cried,
For a morsel of manna begged and tried;
But now thou sleepest, dazed and tired; on cheeks
Undried lie drops of fresh-wept tears
While nectar touches thy lips, - partake,-
Wake, wake my sleeping Hunger, wake!

This unquenched hunger old of mine
Did eat all food and yet did pine,-
Was starved with surfeit and it sought
How might its yearn'd-for food be got.
The food for which thou wept'st awaits, - partake! —
Wake, wake my sleeping Hunger, wake!

Friends and wealth and fancy's rarest treat,
Posthumous wishes sprung from deathless roots so sweet
Did fail to feed thy heart's true crave
And burned with thousand flaming waves
The nectar sought for seeks thee now;-partake —
Wake, wake my sleeping Hunger, wake!

My hunger burned and wept to drink

Songs of the Soul

The mysteries by life's bare brink, -
Ambrosial founts that sleep beneath
The mysteries caves on soil of truth;
Weep more drops, nay streams — ocean-of tears,
Thy duty is for peace to weep; thy only care
To seek thy work; and all thy food
Be what doth nourish thy mood:
Thy work is done, thy nectar's here,-
Quench, quench the eternal ache! —
Wake, wake my sleeping Hunger, wake!


ETERNITY

Oh, will that day arrive
When I shall ceaselessly ask, and drive
Eternal questions
Into Thine ear, O Eternity, and await solution
As to how weak weeds do grow and stand unbent,
Unshak'n beneath the trampling current;
How the storm did wreck titanic things, rooted trees,
And quick disturbed the mighty seas;
How the first spark blinked, and the first tree,
The first goldfish, the first blue bird so free
And the first crooning baby
In this wonder house made their visit and entry.
They come, I see;
Their growth alone I watch;
Thy Cosmic Moulding Hand
That secret works on land and seas
I wish to seize
O Eternity!

## VANISHING BUBBLES

Many unknown bubbles float and flow,
Many ripples dance by me
And melt away in sea.
I like to know, ah, whence they come or whither
go-

The rain drops and dies,
My thoughts play wild and vanish quick,
The red clouds melt in skies:
I stake my purse or slave all life their motive still to seek.

Some friends, though not their love,
Some dearest thoughts I ne'er would lose, I said,
And Last night's surest stars, seen just above,-
All, all are fled.

The crowds of lilies, the linnet,
Perfumed blossoms, honey-mad bees,
Met once on yonder bowered trees;
Now the lonesome field alone is left.

The bubbles, lilies, friends, dramatic thoughts-
They all their part did play and entertain,
And now beneath the grassy screen, to change their displayed
coats,
They quiet, concealed remain.

## VARIETY

I sought for twins
I could not find;
I search my mind,
No twins have seen.

They seem alike,
Man and man, beast and brute
Yet no faces two are like;
Ne'er the same song sang the lute.

Ne'er two hearts are same.
I bow to each new form and name —
Variety complete.
Through forms infinite.

I wish that I were you and he,
And all at once what I would-be;
Oh, could I wear at will all terrene minds,
Like robes of newer kinds!

Then would I flash forth varied smiles
Or languorous walk in sorrow robed,
Or charm with sparkling wiles
And time beguile;

Or march with martial songs,
To right all worldly wrongs;
Or wear a powerful prophet mind
And into dust earth's sorrows grind;

Or wear the youthful hermit's heart,
To scatter love and strength impart.

I'd wear each heart
And don each will and smiles and spend my pelf
To try all noble minds and thoughts
And take what suits myself.

With brain-born nixes,
With marsh-marauding hopes and pixies,
With every elfin thought that timid trod on mind
I'd friendship find.

To soul of the new in things
My spirit homage sings,
I would not taste the same nectar,
Nor twice drink from th' Immortals' jar,

Thy presence, O Eternity,
Show Thou in endless variety!
Yet change not me,
Though various my costumes be.


## THE BLOOD OF ROSE

I tore the rose,
I bled its slender stem,
Its petals quivered
And I shivered;
Yet I dared to rob its smell!

Songs of the Soul

My heart did break and tell,
"Thy hands are soiled," and mute I stood,
Thus self-condemned and stained with rose's blood.
But I know now,
I love the rose
More than its wealth, and vow
Ne'er its love to desecrate or lose.


## AT THE ROOTS OF ETERNITY

With sailing clouds and plunging breeze,
With swaying trees and youthful, stormy seas,
With whirling planets I wildly play
In some absorbing way
But not always;-
At close of day
I lay
My eager hands at the roots of Eternity
To seize and own its nectar free.


## UNDYING BEAUTY

They did their best
And they are blest,-
The sap, the shoots,
The little leaves and root;
The benign breath,
The touch of light,-
All worked in amity
To grow the rose's beauty.

The Essence of Kriya Yoga

Watch its splendor,
Its undying grandeur,
The Infinite Face
That peeps through its little case;-
Watch not in grief
Sojourn here;-
For its career
Done, its duty ends;
Toward the Immortals' home it tends.
The sap dried,
The summer petals fled.
Its body pines;
Yet its death's divine;
Through death and spurns
Its deathless glory won:
The rose is dead,-
Its beauty lives instead.


THE NOBLE NEW

Sing songs that none have sung,
Think thoughts that in brain have never rung'
Walk in paths that none have trod,
Weep tears as none have shed for Lord,
Love all with love that none have felt, and brave
The battle of life with strength unchained,
Give peace to all to whom none other gave,
Claim him your own who is e'er disclaimed.

## PROTECTING THORNS

The charm of the blushing rose
Hides its stinging thorns beneath;
Yet without the wounds from those
Thou could'st not snatch its wealth with stealth,-
The rose with thorns unstained with blood,
The rose that sprang from earthly sod.
In her defense the thorns do sting,
To keep thee out by thorny ring;
Yet the perfumed petals' show
They drowsing soul doth wake and draw;
If thou dost love the beauty alone
Why would'st thou rush to bleed from prickly thorns?

## TATTERED GARMENT

Oh, sing no plaintive lay
When at last my earthly raiment dies,
Nor let ashes tell thy tear where it lies;
Oh, blow my tattered garment's dust away!

The dust clean washed,
The hidden gold beneath will show
Itself anew all bright and brushed,
And shine somewhere aglow,-

And wait with luring luster
For some home-lorn soul
To show the path with lightning glimmer

## The Essence of Kriya Yoga

From darkness on to goal.
IN STILLNESS DARK

Hark!
In stillness dark,
When noisy dreams have slept,
The house is gone to rest,
And busy life
Doth cease from strife,-
The soul in pity soft doth kiss
The truant flesh to soothe, and speak
With mind-transcending grace
Its soundless voice of peace.

Through transient fissures deep
In walls of sleep
Take thou a gentle peep;
Nor droop, nor stare,
But watch with care
The sacred glare,
Ablaze and clear.

In golden glee
Flash past thee
So nigh.
Ashamed, Apollo droops in dread
To see that luster spread
Through boundless reach of sky.

## NATURE'S NATURE

Away, ye muses, all away,
Away with songs of finch and fay,
Away the jaundiced sight
That conflagrates the firefly's light
To bonfire,-
That sets ablaze at once
Your musing's burning lamps;
That ornaments with rhymes
The penury-stricken looks betimes;
That over-clothes the Logic lord
With fancy-swollen words.
Away, the partial love
That 'boldens nature to sit above
Her Maker!

This day I fasten eye-lid doors,
With absence wax my ears,
With languor all congeal my tongue, my touch, my
         tears,-
That I myself may pore
Upon the things behind, ahead
Of the darkness 'round me spread.
I lock Dame Nature out
With all her fickle rout:
Somewhere here
In the darkness drear
I myself with cheer
My course will steer

In the path

## The Essence of Kriya Yoga

E'er sought by all:
Its magnet-call
I hear.

Not here, not here
Apollo would his burning chariot steer;
Nor Dian dares to peep
Into the sacred silence deep.

Nor here, not here
The mounts nor rebel waves, nor far or near,
Can make me full of fear, nor evermore
Their dreadful grandeur adore.

Not here, not here
The soft capricious wiles of flowers,
Nor swarming storm clouds' sweeping terror,
Nor doomsday's thunder roar
Dismantling earth and stars,
The cosmic beauties all to mar;

Dishevelling of trees
And light-hearted skies,
Nor nature's murderous mutiny
Nor man's exploding destiny
Can touch me here.

Nor here, not here-
Through mind's strong iron bars
No gods nor goblins, no men nor nature
Without my pass dare enter.
I look behind, ahead,

Songs of the Soul

And on naught but darkness tread,
In wrath I strike, and set it ablaze
With the immortal spark of thought,
By the friction-process brought
Of concentration
And distraction;-
The darkness burns
With a million tongues,
And now I spy
All past, all distant things as nigh.

I smile serene
As I expose to gaze
In wisdom's brilliant blaze
All charms of the Hidden Home Unseen:
The Home of Nature's birth,
The planets' moulding hearth,
The factory whence all forms of fairies start,
The bards, colossal minds and hearts,
The gods and all,
And all, and all!

Away, Away
With all the lightsome lays;-
Oh, I'll now portray
In humble way,
And try t lisp half-truths
Of wordless charms of The Unseen
To whom Nature her nature owes, and sheen.

The Essence of Kriya Yoga

## MY KINSMEN

In spacious hall of trance I spied –
Aglow with million dazzling lights,
Tapestried with the snowy cloud –
My kinsmen all, lowly, proud;

The banquet great with music rolls,
The drum of Om[1] in measure falls,
The hosts, in many ways arrayed,
Some plain, some gorgeous dress displayed.

Around the various tables large
Of earth and moon and sun and stars,
The countless mute, and noisy guests
Observed Dame Nature's feast with zest.

The tiny-eyed and shiny sands,
Thirsty, drank of ocean's life:
I well remember once I brawled
For a sip of sea, with kinsmen sands.

Yes, I know those old dame rocks
Who rocked me on their stony laps
When I a tiny baby tree
Did chafe to run with winds so free.

[1]Cosmic Vibration

Songs of the Soul

The green-attired friends I know,
With rose and lily buds aglow;
I once adorned a kingly breast,
Lost life, returned to mother dust.

I know the ruby redbreast dear,
My blood in it once flowed so clear;
I smiled in diamonds, gleaming bright,
I danced in Roentgen rays of light.

A ray of friendship from my heart
In diamond and ruby joy did start,
The bright ones smiled, the ruby wept
To meet their long-lost friend at last.

The soul of gold in yellow gown,
The soul of silver whitely shone,-
Bestowed on me maternal smiles
That told they knew me long erewhile.

The lark, the cuckoo, the pheasant sweet,
The deer, the lamb, the lion great,
The shark and monsters of the sea!
In love and peace all greeted me.

The leafy fingers, arms outspread,
Caressed me when a tiny bird,
And fed me with ambrosial fruit
That drew its life from immortal root.

When atoms and the star-dust sprang,
When Vedas, Bible, Koran sang,-

## The Essence of Kriya Yoga

I joined each choir; their long-past thrilling songs
Still echo in my soul in accents strong.


## OM

Whence, Oh, this soundless roar doth come
When drowseth matter's dreary drum?-
The booming Om on bliss shore breaks;
All heaven all earth, all body shakes.

Cords bound to flesh are broken all,
Vibrations vile do fly and fall;
The hustling heart, the boasting breath
No more disturb the yogi's health.

The house is lulled in darkness soft,
Dim, shiny light is seen aloft,
Subconscious dreams have gone to bed.
'Tis then that one doth hear Om's tread.

The bumble bee doth hum along,
Baby Om, hark! Sings his song:
Krishna's flute is sounding sweet,
'Tis time the watery God to meet:
God of fire is now singing
Om, - Om — his harp is ringing;
God of prana[2] is now sounding,
Wondrous bell of soul resounding.

[2]Vibration of life energy

Songs of the Soul

Upward climb the living tree,
Hear the sound of ethereal sea;
Marching mind doth homeward hie
To join the Christmas Symphony.

## MYSTERY

Burst, inky cloud, do burst,
Fling open thy fathomless gloom!
In Thy dark chamber must
A million mysteries loom.

Heartless, staring sky!
Make quick reply
To aching query of my straining eye,
Show what thou hidest and why;-
The ceaseless surging thoughts
Go mocking, dancing by,
I long to know their lot.
Someone did throw me free
To battle all alone in this rough sea.
Rudderless I drift,
Stranded on shoals my boat couldn't shift.
I'll burst the clouds, I'll clean the shoals,
I'll rip the sky in twain,
I'll break my heart,
With question crush my brain-
I'll ask and pray,
Will beg or steal
To find the friends long stolen away,
To know their woe or weal.

The Essence of Kriya Yoga

This wondrous day,
Stage set for play
By Unseen Hand,-
The players drop
From no-man's land,
Then vanish away or stop
With changing scenes of birth and death.
The drama's on
The actors play anon
Yet know not why they play
This glorious day!


IT"S ALL UNKNOWN

Each rose-bud dawning day,
In hourly opening petal-rays
    Doth fair display
    Its hidden beauty.

The petal-hours, unfolding smile,
My drooping, lagging heart beguile
Day spreads its petals all
Of novel hopes and joys withal.
    The rose-buds' there, -
    "Today" is here;
In time the rose-bud blooms, -
While lazy day oft glooms.
    Forsake thy sleep
    O, Lazy Day,
Open Thou with thy full-bloom ray
To chase my gathered gloom away!

The rose-bud opened,
The day now smiled
In fullness fine;
Still I opine
'Tis all unknown
Just why the rose was blown,
And the day was drowned in night
Then raised again to light
Of glorious dawn,
So swiftly marching o'er the lawn!


SILENCE

The earth, the planets play
In and through the sun-born rays
In majesty profound.
Umpire Time
In silence sublime
Doth watch
This cosmic match.

The Author of the great game
Assumes no spoken name;-
With boundless poise
He doth His will without a noise,
Ungrateful moods ignoring,
Unkindness all forgiving.

Truth clearly speaks to all,
But speaks not loud;
They hear its call

The Essence of Kriya Yoga

Who noise enthrall.

The voice in threatening silence speaks
To those who error's path do seek.
The tiger may be tamed,
Failures' talons can be maimed,
Unruly nature trained
By powerful silence o' unspoken words,
If in Truth maintained.


AT THE FOUTAIN OF SONG

Dig, dig, yet deeper dig
In the stony earth for fount of song
Dig, dig yet deeper dig
In soil of muse's heart along.

Some sparkle is seen,
Some bubble is heard;
'T is then unseen,-
The bubble is dead.

The watery sheen
Again doth show:
Dig, Dig still deeper e'en
Till the bubble song again would grow.

I hear the song,
I see its body bright,-
Yet cannot touch-I long
To seize it now and drink its liquid light.

Songs of the Soul

Bleed, O my Soul, do amply bleed
To dig yet deeper,-dig!

I touch the holy fount, - rejoice,
I drink its bubble voice
My throat's ablaze,-
I want to drink and drink always;
The sphere's aflame
With my thirst as I came:
So dig, dig, yet deeper dig
Though it seems thou canst not dig!

I thought with heart aglow
All, all, I had drunk this day,
And idly looked for more, deep, deep, below,-
But lo! Undrunk, untouched,
There the fountain lay.


THE EVER NEW

Newer joys adorn the day,
Brighter burn through livelong night
The stars with purer light,
Brighter thoughts do brace my voice,
Newer words await my choice,
With heart of th' new I'll sing my lay-
Wings of thoughts would ceaseless beat
The sky of time, and race to meet
Thy distant throne
That somewhere is alone.

The Essence of Kriya Yoga

Each and every day
Men choir some song
Not with thoughts the same but a changing
Throng
Of newer ones that make Thy greater lay-

The bubbling joy
Of each little boy,
Each brew of friendship still
I steal, and with them fill
Mine cup of ageless heart
With ceaseless thrills to start.
Morrow each and each today
With newer love I'll sing my lay,
The voices same do sing the lay
In temple church and fane:
But I deign ne'er to hear
The strains all stained with age-old tear;
My fountain flows anew today,
With newer tears will flow my lay.
In the same old church
I'll newly sing and search,
In the same old sermon
For unending truths and newer reason;
In the same old organ will I seek
The newer hopes of new-born week.

Every day, oh, every day
The bell will ring a new Sunday,
And bathed in Thy beaming ray
With newer thoughts I'll sing my lay.

## THE EVER-TRODDEN PATH

This ever-trodden path
Where travelers all of earth
Do walk in joyous haste
Or slothful sorrow's state
I walk and wonder,-
In truth or blunder.
The path is cleft
To right and left,
In front, behind,-
The diverse ways I find,
Bewildered am I —
As baffling mazes do they lie;
    Still, they say
    There's a royal way
For all-the right, the error-wed,-
    'Tis the sub-way path of ruby red
    Which far beneath lies hid
    For eager eyes to lead
    Straight on the feet
To where all paths do meet.


## THE HUMAN MIND

I love to roam alone, unseen,
In cities of the human mind.
Untrodden by the crooked thoughts
    Vile-born, -unkind.

Incognito I wish to wander,

## The Essence of Kriya Yoga

To living lanes my thoughts surrender
With simple wish to know and learn
The straight nice paths and danger turns.

I wish to roam in mazy lanes
Of dark and brighter thoughts,
With love to all and harm to none,
With better message fraught.

I'd love to broaden narrow lanes
Of selfish crooked thoughts
With my love's true-building brain
That I've within me got.

I long to soar so high
That I at once may spy
The narrow alleys, broader roads
Of human thoughtful moods.


## THE CUP OF ETERNITY

The traveler of the endless track
All weary, thirsty, sore doth seek
To quench the quenchless mortal thirst,
The wordless worry of his heart.
He spies a cup-a little orb,
He tries to drink with joyful sob,
He stands aback, the cup sets down,-
On the contents scant his heart did frown.

Yet up he lifts the cup again,

Songs of the Soul

But fears his baneful thirst to flame.
When, hark! A voice of counsel deep
Forbids him this to soil with lip.

The cup so small to mortal eye,-
The cup whose depth the wise can spy
Dries up, alas! If mortals drink;
Perennial fount, the soulful think.

Now, in the little cup he'll see
The sunsounded deep of eternity;
For ageless hours and endless days
The ambrosial drink he'll taste and praise.

The deathly thirst so fleshly born
Ne'er shall parch his soul again;
The cup he'll drink, but not the bane
To quench his thirst, and bliss attain.
And vain would mighty north winds try
Compassion's gathered tears to dry.


A MIRROR NEW

I bring to you
A mirror new-
A glass of introspection clear,
That illusions shows and sooty fear
That spots thy mind.
Thou wilt find
This mirror new
        Would also show all true

The Essence of Kriya Yoga

The "Inner You,"
That's veiled in flesh
And doth ne'er appear.
Each night consult afresh
Thy mirror friend and clear away
The dust that gathers each day.


THE SPELL

Ah, this old, old nectar of night
Brewed below by sun God bright1-
Let every little fleshly cell
That's tired and thirsty drink it well.
By soothing spell of sleep eject
All aches that heart and brain infect!
The spell quick marching on
Falls on me now so warm,
And robs my mind
Of linked thoughts, to bind
Me prisoner in its charm.

## MY NATIVE LAND

The friendly sky,
Inviting shades of banian tree,
The holy Ganges flowing by,-
How can I forget thee!

I love the waving corn
Of India's fields so bright,
Oh, better than those Heav'nly grown
By deathless gods of might.

My soul's broad love so grand
Was born here first below,-
In my own native land,
On India's sunny soil aglow.

I love thy breeze,
I love thy moon,
I love thy hills and seas,
In thee I wish to cease, or swoon.

Thou taught'st me first to love
Thy sky, the stars, the God above;
So my first homage meets,
O India, at thy feet!
From thee I now have learn'd to see,
To love all lands alike as thee;
I bow to thee, my native land,
The Mother of my love so grand.

## ON COMING TO THE NEW-OLD LAND-AMERICA

Sleeping memories
Of friends once more to be
Did greet me – sailing o'er the sea,-
     Sensing my coming
The Pilgrim Lad to adore,
The distant sleeping shore
Lay in the twinkling night,
Dim throught the vanished light,
     The breeze wafted strong
       Strange thoughts
    That my brain did throng,
      Hopes sweet and richly wrought.

The raven-winged gloom did perch
On the portals of my mind and search
My soul, my strength to awe;
     Yet crowds with joy oh, then, I saw

Of phantom friends
Now come to lend
Their cheer,
And end my fear!


## THE TOILER'S LAY

From school of life,
From bossy duty's binding day,
From hours of dollar-strife
I wish I were a run-away!

Songs of the Soul

From chasing worry hound
I'll fly one day,
From crowds and throngs around
I wish I were a run-away!

From greedy food
That steals its way,
From luring dainties' tempting mood
I wish I were a run-away!

From homely cups and chairs and couch
The call of grassy-bed today
My heart doth snatch;-
I wish I were a run-away!

From nature's given cup,
My hollow hands, I'l drink
At the streamlet's bounteous brink;
With finger forks I'll eat the meat
Of fresh plucked fruits from trees, my seat
All snug beneath the shady trees,
Enliv'n'd by birds and bumble bees,
Fanned by mothering air,
From care and tear
I'll bathe my weary mind
In new-made joyous day;
Away dish-washing, cups and saucers, all away!
For just a day
I wish I were a run-away!

## CITY DRUM

'Tis morn
The rolling wheels are on
Of a marching world
So strong.

I love to be roused
From a silent sleep
By the early hum
Of the active city drum.

The drum beats
To loudly greet
All those heroes true
That would die or do, -
To meet the morning's foe
Of worry or of woe
With a dauntless smile,
And thus success beguile
Unto the happy camp
Where peace e'er burns its lmap.
The city's drum
With its noisy hum
Announces true and strong
The world is marching on.

## MOHAWK TRAIL

Welcomed by a fresh and smiling day,
Usher'd by trees benign that lay
To shade our bodies from the jealous sun,
With rubber shoes pressing on asphalt road,
With softly humming noise we rode
Through Mohawk Trail where Adam lies
Unlike all other joyful rides
When mind with sameness was dulled sometimes and
      did abide
The time and common scenes in passive mood,
My mind was now so full, bright and good.
A strange, unknown, unthought, new thrill
Did steal o'er me in soothing sweep so still.
I raced with wind and scattered smiles
That played with sunshine, spread for miles.
My secret hoarded joy in vault of soul
I extravagantly did spend withal
To buy new nature's gaudy scenes
That one hasty, racing peddler brought me in.
My spirit hemm'd in city's narrow walls
Was free once more; all nature sent a joyous call;
The waving leaves of trees, the babbling rill,
The impatient wind, smiling skies and hill.

PIKE'S PEAK

Ne're did I expect to roam
On wheels four
Where thousand clouds do soar.
The dangerous darksome path
With "W" winding tricky curves that climbed
And in secret glided
Fourteen thousand feet above the sea
In the home of darky clouds, so gamesome free
That watched with heavy binding vapour-shroud
To cast around strange steps
That dared to tread in stealth
Their home of scenic wealth.
And I did swoon
To spy in the light of the miser moon
The deep, deep hollow hall of vacant space below
Dimly 'dorned with weird light
Pictures of twinkling, sleeping cities, shadowy trees,
          valleys bright.
Resting breezes, leaves and tall soldiers – stones
Meantime the dim moonlight
Was slowly, strangely changing into light of dawn.
There is the temple observatory
Vacant and solitary.
Alas! Where are Thy swarming lovers
O Royal Phoebus
As blushing red thou didst burn
In the earliest hour of dawn?
The testing, biting chill
Drove all Thy votaries away
And all was still

Songs of the Soul

And I was left alone
With Thee. Thou wert aflame
Yet calmer now
With a silvery brow
Spreading o'er sleeping creatures
To wake them
They did awake
The trees breathed
And the streamlets opened their crystal, twinkling eyes
All creation rose from sleep.
I know
O Redeemer of Darkness now.
All waked-up creatures, things
Looking in wonder
Not at thee but at the Unseen Wonder
Whom thou dost thru thy glow
Mutely want to show.
Where was the cold?
Rebuked it fled, the troublesome chill of old.
I loved the breathless subtle air
So pure and clear
That chokes the gross
And burns the dross
Of those that love
To worship Thee in breathless state, O far above
The roar and din
Of tipsy senses.
I met all minds,
I asked the winds,
I pursued the rainbow,
I begged the pure white clouds
Which sailed unknown so proud

The Essence of Kriya Yoga

To tell me if they saw
Whom I just spied;
Whose One Face to see I tried
Midst bewitching, bewildering, diverse crowds
Of scenic faces, and I cried aloud
To see Him hide
Beneath the beauty tide.


PAUPAC'S PEAK

Paupac's Peak
With rustic scenes and trees
I found and seek
In thee some Hidden Beauties,
Thy palace I entered
Thru thy woody road
Where both ways stood thy columned trees with
        leafy swords
Outstretched, and a bowered welcome rendered.
Unconscious hopes and thrill
To know thy royal mysteries still
And tempted was I
Thy secrets to pry.
I stole thru secret hilly ways.
And all at once stood face to face
Where thy liquid silver spray did grace
The breast of caves and down did run
Sparkling thru rays of sun
To ornament the crude stones and logs beneath
With eddying necklace and pearly bubbled wreath.
There I tore thru

Songs of the Soul

The veil of trees and spied
All sudden Thy peaceful Paupac, and in wonder cried
To find on cloudy breast of proud high hills
Myriad tears all closely gathered still
Into a lake
All ready to be kind to me and slake
My parching thirst of mind
The Unseen Strength to find.

The cool breeze was wooing the lake's warm waters
In hidden snow-white mist
That didn't resist
Two leafy canoe vessels
Laden with silhouettes of singing angels across the sky,
Swimming like peaceful swans
At farewell hour of the sun.
Once I entered a covered path inlaid
With velvet moss and sunshine-checkered cushion of
        leaves who gave
Their silken bodies up for all to tread
And dance in comfort waves
Could wealth audacious e'er dare to make
Such bowered unfading garland of the lake
Of countless rhododendrons
That in summer
With white and pink flowers
The woodland darkness adorn?
I passed thru these corridors of trees
Who tries to hide with their finger-leaves
The sparkling beauty of the lake on left.
Of cares bereft
I walked by this garland path

The Essence of Kriya Yoga

And many a time in wrath
I would command
My noisy footsteps and thoughts in stillness to stand.
And I did bow in sweetest reverence
To the spirit in this temple of silence.
I stood still and gazed within, without,
At the thoughts, the feelings, leaves, stones, my body,
        skies, earth and light.
But wherever I saw
Thy tender Peeping Eyes my soul did draw.


SCENES WITHIN

Wondrous scenic faces
The Denver horizon graces.
Yet when I think of the better beauties
That lie in human souls
Rapture calls.
Then eager I look
And delve deep in the valleys
Of human minds and their sacred nooks,
Colossal mounts of nobility
Adorned with every quality
I find there,
Marigold, rose and pure white flowers
Of budding thoughts
With growing perfumes attract.
There's the blue expanse of amity
With ripples of thrill and endless beauty.
Perpetual freshness of soul and constant kind looks
Down do flow the mountain bosom like brooks.

Songs of the Soul

Matchless founts of love
Bubble forth in the heart
Of this garden of soul, and start
Endless sparkling fancies.
There in the land of souls
Blow the various breezes.
Some warm  me, some freeze;
Warm souls, vital souls
Breathe the living air in me
My doors are open wide and free

I open my eyes and pass
By the mountain scenes,
Now I close my eyes
And race in my mind's aerial plane
Viewing the unseen garden of souls
Cities of passions all,
Liquid, mazy desires,
Deceiving mires,
Ego's dark titanic chasms
Where faith ne'er shone.
What Lands I pass?
Whose kingdom I see?
There, there alone I find
Real America
Or living India,
There I see the beauties and the barren tracts
Of nations all and minds all,
Yet various tho this Kingdom be
Lives there but One Beauty.

Three thousand miles of tracts I traveled not

The Essence of Kriya Yoga

But thru three thousand miles of minds was I
Brought,
I find writ
And well knit
In the scenes, fields, garden and shops
The vibrations and thoughts of minds and of cities.
Many pass unheeding the beauties
Of their familiar paths and trees;
Many roam in the garden of hearts
In blindness.
Thus I long to start
In them a vision new
Of beauty eternal and true.


## THE GRAND CANYON OF THE COLORADO

Who reigns in this Canyon
Deep and grand with measureless space?
The Sun or Moon?
Who in jealousy vie
To drive away in swiftness
The demon of darkness
And try
To wake the sleeping motley colors
And splendor
To decorate in glory
The crowded temple peaks both young and hoary
Who though different yet in unison
Do welcome all to see the One.

The temple of Siva and Rama

Songs of the Soul

In silence worship the one Brahma.
Who reigns here?
To inspire
All eyes, all minds, all sects, all creeds,
To suit their all aesthetic needs
And make them in awe and reverence
Bow to the Spirit of Vastness that here reigns.


## LIFE'S DREAM
Dedicated to
The Mount Washington Educational Center, Los Angeles,
Headquarters of Yogoda and Sat-Sanga.


The summer-East
And the wintry West
They say-but Mount Washington
Named rightly after that pioneer,
Of Freedom's great career,
Thou dost stand, the snowless guardian Himalaya
Of the angel land in perpetual green regalia.
Nippon's camphor trees and perfumed wisteria and
          smiling roses
Palm, date and well-beloved spicy bay leaves of Hind
          stand close,
With endless scenic beauties
Of ocean, canyon, setting sun, moon-studded sky
And nightly twinkling cities
To declare
Thy ever-changing beauty.
On thy crown thou shalt newly wear
A priceless starry-school which in all future near

Shall draw the lost travelers of the East and West
To find their goal and one place of rest.
Here one path
Shall merge with all other paths.
Here the love of earthly Freedom's paradise, America,
Shall blend fore'er with spiritual Freedom's paradise,
        India.
Here church in deepest friendliness shall other churches
        meet,
Here the temple the mosque shall greet.
Here the long-divorced matter-laws
Will wed again in peace the spirit-laws.
Here all minds will learn that true Art
Of living life and the way to start
Straight to the One great place
Where all must meet at last.
Jehovah! This is the land of solace
Where my life's dream in truth reappears!


## LUTHER BURBANK

Beatific Burbank
The great reformer Luther thou art
Of living plants and flowers
(Of all moods,
The tender ones, the stubborn growing ones,
Or the cactus rude).
Thy peaceful ways
The cruel cactus took
And its armored thorns forsook
And learned to sacrifice its meat

Songs of the Soul

For all to eat.
Ten score years the hard-shelled stubborn walnut tree
Took to fully grow-
Thy care did soften its shell and taught it nine score years
to throw.
The flower-smile on thy face
Tells thou art nurtured on Nature's green breast bedecked
with petal' lace.
Soul met soul so free
And I saw thee
A God-grown mental lotus-flower
Just opening tender
Not only to cast the beauty rays
Of thy plant knowledge and its supreme ways
To your fellow man,
But also gently turning to the Mighty Invisible sun
That lights little plants, distant stars, the bursting
bubble, thee and me and man.
Thou didst not ask, "Who thou art?"
But understood my speaking heart,
Our souls touched and we saw
We had but one goal, one task, one law,
By knowledge to break
The walls of dogma dark.

On the ocean's surface is diversity
Beneath lies all the waves in One Unity.
We both dived deep-
Thou thru living waves of plants
And I thru waves of human minds.
We found we meet beneath
(As all deep divers do

# The Essence of Kriya Yoga

On a vast expanse of Unity)
In this great Truth-Sea.

Thou dost dread isms and dogmas
So do I all man-made false enigmas.
We outcasts know but one bright
Truth-made path of light.
God didst make thee and all in His image,
Certs thou hast broken the dogmas of age
By creating new fruits, new plants,
And  shown the world in wonder
The Creator's child too a creator,
> We go not in
> That's why we say
> "He's far away, O far away."
> He dost not hid from us
> But we from him.
> Let's rush
> Within let's go
> Lo!
> He's there always.

O Santa Rosa
Blest thou art to have blown
The perfume of thy one great flower
For distant people of the earth to enjoy its shower
Of scent so sweet.
If Nature makes some imperfect plant,
Burbank by his magic wand
Its invading germs disbands.
Or creates new kinds
With new coats, quickened in age and color.-

## Songs of the Soul

There's a suggestion for you, dear world,
That his life imparts.-
If weak, afflicted, or error-fixed thou art,
Thou canst (if thy reason starts
In the direction right
With determined might
To become all free)
Be what thy soul wishes and works to be.
Santa Rosa, thy flower the ages shall not fade,
In the soil of memories ever-fresh it shall live endless
            decades.

FOREWORD

The eleventh chapter of the Bhagavadgita, of which "Vision of Visions" is a lyrical rendition interwoven with an interpretation of its spiritual significance, is the consummation of the teachings of the Book. It describes how the Lord Krishna, the Warrior-Prophet, blessed Arjuna, his devotee, with the great yogic vision of the cosmic drama of life and death, enacted on the Infinite Body of the Lord by Himself. Arjuna, still human, was perplexed, being unable reconcile the benign aspect of the Lord with His destructive aspect: doing good to men and the world as a whole on the one hand, and bringing death and destruction to countless creatures and worlds on the other. It has been shown here that life and death are both momentary scenes in the cosmic drama, meant not to hurt or please anybody, but designed to afford infinite opportunities to the Lord's children for the attainment of higher and higher states of evolution through apparently unpleasant disturbances caused by great changes. The relative value of life and death in this Drama, which is a dream in comparison with the Reality of the Lord, is the same. This vision represents the great Cosmic Law, as seen not from the point of view of finite creatures, but from that of the Lord Himself. Hence this allows no room for the finite questioning of Arjuna as to whether the Lord is benign or destructive. To Him, to destroy life is not an absence of us. The Lord view life and death as forms of change only, according to His Cosmic Law. A law is law. It has been His nature, and always will be. There is no question about benignity or otherwise.

Nevertheless, it describes the Lord as leading this Cosmos with all its individuals to higher and higher stages of unfoldment.

Every individual is expected to do his duty unattached, with the consciousness of an intelligent agent merely, that he can reach those higher stages easily, and finally be in tune with that Great Being.

## VISION OF VISIONS

Arjuna said:
"Beloved Lord,
Adored of gods,
Behold, behold
Thy body holds
All fleshly tenants, seers fine,
The diverse saints divine.
      Dwelling deep in mystery cave,
The Serpent Nature's forceful crave,
Though fierce and subtle, now is tame,
Forgetful of her deadly game;
And Sovran Brahma, God of gods,
On lotus seat is snug secured.
O Cosmic-Bodied Lord of worlds,
Oh, I behold, again behold
Thee all and everywhere
Thy countless arms and trunks and eyes!
Yet, drooping dark my knowledge lies
About Thy birth and reign and presence here.
This day,
O Blazing, Furious Flame,
O Blinding Ray,
Thy focused power's aglow: Thy Name
Spreads everywhere
To dark'st abysmal lair.
Thou, gilded with a crown of stars,
And wielding mace of sovereign power,
Thou whirlest forth, O Burning Phoebus,
Thy evolution's circling discus.
Immortal Brahma, all Supreme,

Songs of the Soul

Thou Cosmic Shelter, Wisdom's Theme,
Eternal Dharma's[3] guardian true,
Thou diest not I ever knew!

O Birthless, Fleshless, Deathless One,
Unseen, thy endless, working arms,
Thy Ever-Watching Eyes!
The suns and moons and staring skies,
Thy Selfborn Lustre shields from harm,
And the distant creation warms.
O Sovereign Soul, this earth and gods.
All high-abodes and all encircling spheres,
Directions all, and earthly sods,
By Thee pervaded, far and near,
And worldly beings, struck by fear,
Thy wondrous form adore.

In Thee the gods their entry make
With folded hands, afraid, some pray to shelter take
In Thee. The seers great, on Heaven's path successful ones,
With superb hymns of peace do worship Thee and
        Thee alone.
The eleven lamps of Heaven,
The twelve bright suns,
The grizzly Eight,
The starry lustres great,
Aspiring hermits, gods,
The agents of the Cosmic Lord,

[3]Religion or Self-Expression

118

## The Essence of Kriya Yoga

The twin-born princes strong,
Of valor known so long,
Two-score and nine noil breezes' force,
That binds the atoms close,
The long-passed guardian spirits all,
The demi-goblins, gods and demons tall,
Mighty ones in Spirit's path,
In wonder all behold Thy blazoned worth.
I Thee behold
Colossal-armed, with countless cheeks,
And starry eyes, with endless hands, and legs adorned
With lotus feet.
Thy chasmed mouth, with doomsday's teeth
Doth yawn to swallow swooning worlds around,
And leaves a distilled joyous awe in me.
Thy grandeur I and all are wonder-struck to see.
The bowels of the void deep are filled with Thee
Thy diverse hues and gaping mouths and luster-smeared
body,
O Vishnu[4] of the flaming sight,
Thou now awest me, my peace dost fright.
Ferocious teeth and deadly fires do howl
In mouths of Thine which at me scowl.

Directions four are lost and gone,
I find no peace alone.
Cosmic Guardian, Lord of gods,
Be pleased t' accept my humble words.

[4]The Great Spirit

Songs of the Soul

The Ego, Karma, Senses great abide
And wait to leap upon our Wisdom's chiefs.
And yet thy both do ride
The race of death, to fall and hide
For e'er in thy devouring mouth,
Adorned with crushing cruel teeth uncouth.

The victor and the vanquished must,
(Thy offsprings both, the righteous and ungodly ones,)
Thy love still claim, yet all some day shall kiss the dust,
And sleep on common color of earth.
The shattered  skulls of some are seen,
As caught Thy greedy teeth between.

As diverse, restless, watery waves
Of river branches all do crave
To force through crowded wavelets' way,
And meet where Neptune's home long lay,
So the heroic streams of life
Do plunge to meet in maddest strife
At Thy foaming mouth of sea,
Where sparkling lives do dance so free:
As insects lost in beauty's game
All swiftly, thoughtless rush to flame,
So fog-born passion's fires pretend
To glow like Heav'nly light of Thine,
And draw on mortals to attend
The trumpet call to deathly line.
Thy mouth ablaze
Doth bring to gaze
Its leaping tongues to lick
The angry blood of strong and weak.

## The Essence of Kriya Yoga

Thou Gourmand God dost eat
With hunger Infinite;
O Vishnu, Thou dost scorch
The worlds with all-pervading fiery torch.

Be please, O Prime of gods;
I ache to know Thee, Primeval Lord.
O tell, Thou, O Fiery Mood,
Who art yet so good,-
Thy Royal Will,
I know not still."
The Lord sang:
"Am Endless Doom,
Ready to room
In burning maw
Of mine the weaklings' awe
And all the mortal meat
Of weary worlds of deathly change, and treat
Them with my nectar life
To new and fearless, better strife.
E'en if thou dost not slay
These wicked warriors all in war array
They surely certain have to fall,
Ah, in my teeth-of-law, withal,
Arise, awake! Arise, awake!
Oh, dash to war thy foe, the flesh a captive make,
And seize the victor's fame,
With battle-hunted game,
Wealth of the King
Of Peace, and Heaven's Kingdom bring.
I know right now the happenings all
Which mystic future forth doth call,

And thus thy foes and warriors true,
Long, long ago I slew
Ere thy agent-hand,
That I would wield to land
Thy foes on death's dim shore, could understand.
My agent thou,
Oh, this is how
I work my plans in universe
Through instruments diverse;
'Tis I who slew and yet will slay the senses' train
Through thee, as through both past and future ones,
my soldiers sane."

# Master of Kriya Yoga

## Excerpts from "Autobiography of a Yogi"

Yogananda's Experiences with Sri Yukteswar

## CHAPTER 10

## *I Meet My Master, Sri Yukteswar*

"Faith in God can produce any miracle except one-passing an examination without study." Distastefully I closed the book I had picked up in an idle moment.

"The writer's exception shows his complete lack of faith," I thought. "Poor chap, he has great respect for the midnight oil!"

My promise to Father had been that I would complete my high school studies. I cannot pretend to diligence. The passing months found me less frequently in the classroom than in secluded spots along the Calcutta bathing *ghats*. The adjoining crematory grounds, especially gruesome at night, are considered highly attractive by the yogi. He who would find the Deathless Essence must not be dismayed by a few unadorned skulls. Human inadequacy becomes clear in the gloomy abode of miscellaneous bones. My midnight vigils were thus of a different nature from the scholar's.

The week of final examinations at the Hindu High School was fast approaching. This interrogatory period, like the sepulchral haunts, inspires a well-known terror. My mind was nevertheless at peace. Braving the ghouls, I was exhuming a knowledge not found in lecture halls. But it lacked the art of Swami Pranabananda, who easily appeared in two places at one time. My educational dilemma was plainly a matter for the Infinite Ingenuity. This was my reasoning, though to many it seems illogic. The devotee's irrationality springs from a thousand inexplicable demonstrations of God's instancy in trouble.

"Hello, Mukunda! I catch hardly a glimpse of you these days!" A classmate accosted me one afternoon on Gurpar Road.

"Hello, Nantu! My invisibility at school has actually placed me there in a decidedly awkward position." I unburdened myself under his friendly gaze.

Nantu, who was a brilliant student, laughed heartily; my predicament was not without a comic aspect.

"You are utterly unprepared for the finals! I suppose it is up to me to help you!"

The simple words conveyed divine promise to my ears; with alacrity I visited my friend's home. He kindly outlined the solutions to various problems he considered likely to be set by the instructors.

"These questions are the bait which will catch many trusting boys in the examination trap. Remember my answers, and you will escape without injury."

The night was far gone when I departed. Bursting with unseasoned erudition, I devoutly prayed it would remain for the next few critical days. Nantu had coached me in my various subjects but, under press of time, had forgotten my course in Sanskrit. Fervently I reminded God of the oversight.

I set out on a short walk the next morning, assimilating my new knowledge to the rhythm of swinging footsteps. As I took a short cut through the weeds of a corner lot, my eye fell on a few loose printed sheets. A triumphant pounce proved them to be Sanskrit verse. I sought out a pundit for aid in my stumbling interpretation. His rich voice filled the air with the edgeless, honeyed beauty of the ancient tongue.[1]

"These exceptional stanzas cannot possibly be of aid in your Sanskrit test." The scholar dismissed them skeptically.

But familiarity with that particular poem enabled me on the following day to pass the Sanskrit examination. Through the discerning help Nantu had given, I also attained the minimum grade for success in all my other subjects.

Father was pleased that I had kept my word and concluded my secondary school course. My gratitude sped to the Lord, whose sole guidance I perceived in my visit to Nantu and my walk by the unhabitual route of the debris-filled lot. Playfully He had given a dual expression to His timely design for my rescue.

I came across the discarded book whose author had denied God precedence in the examination halls. I could not restrain a chuckle at my own silent comment:

"It would only add to this fellow's confusion, if I were to tell him that divine meditation among the cadavers is a short cut to a high school diploma!"

In my new dignity, I was now openly planning to leave home. Together with a young friend, Jitendra Mazumdar,[2] I decided to join a Mahamandal hermitage in Benares, and receive its spiritual discipline.

A desolation fell over me one morning at thought of separation from my family. Since Mother's death, my affection had grown especially tender for my two younger brothers, Sananda and Bishnu. I rushed to my retreat, the little attic which had witnessed so many scenes in my turbulent *sadhana*.[3] After a two-hour flood of tears, I felt singularly transformed, as by some alchemical cleanser. All attachment[4] disappeared; my resolution to seek God as the Friend of friends set like granite within me. I quickly completed my travel preparations.

"I make one last plea." Father was distressed as I stood before him for final blessing. "Do not forsake me and your grieving brothers and sisters."

"Revered Father, how can I tell my love for you! But even greater is my love for the Heavenly Father, who has given me the gift of a perfect father on earth. Let me go, that I someday return with a more divine understanding."

With reluctant parental consent, I set out to join Jitendra, already in Benares at the hermitage. On my arrival the young head swami,

Dyananda, greeted me cordially. Tall and thin, of thoughtful mien, he impressed me favorably. His fair face had a Buddhalike composure.

I was pleased that my new home possessed an attic, where I managed to spend the dawn and morning hours. The ashram members, knowing little of meditation practices, thought I should employ my whole time in organizational duties. They gave me praise for my afternoon work in their office.

"Don't try to catch God so soon!" This ridicule from a fellow resident accompanied one of my early departures toward the attic. I went to Dyananda, busy in his small sanctum overlooking the Ganges.

"Swamiji,[5] I don't understand what is required of me here. I am seeking direct perception of God. Without Him, I cannot be satisfied with affiliation or creed or performance of good works."

The orange-robed ecclesiastic gave me an affectionate pat. Staging a mock rebuke, he admonished a few near-by disciples. "Don't bother Mukunda. He will learn our ways."

I politely concealed my doubt. The students left the room, not overly bent with their chastisement. Dyananda had further words for me.

"Mukunda, I see your father is regularly sending you money. Please return it to him; you require none here. A second injunction for your discipline concerns food. Even when you feel hunger, don't mention it."

Whether famishment gleamed in my eye, I knew not. That I was hungry, I knew only too well. The invariable hour for the first hermitage meal was twelve noon. I had been accustomed in my own home to a large breakfast at nine o'clock.

The three-hour gap became daily more interminable. Gone were the Calcutta years when I could rebuke the cook for a ten-minute delay. Now I tried to control my appetite; one day I undertook a twenty-four hour fast. With double zest I awaited the following midday.

"Dyanandaji's train is late; we are not going to eat until he arrives." Jitendra brought me this devastating news. As gesture of welcome to the swami, who had been absent for two weeks, many delicacies were in readiness. An appetizing aroma filled the air. Nothing else offering, what else could be swallowed except pride over yesterday's achievement of a fast?

"Lord hasten the train!" The Heavenly Provider, I thought, was hardly included in the interdiction with which Dyananda had silenced me. Divine Attention was elsewhere, however; the plodding clock covered the hours. Darkness was descending as our leader entered the door. My greeting was one of unfeigned joy.

"Dyanandaji will bathe and meditate before we can serve food." Jitendra approached me again as a bird of ill omen.

I was in near-collapse. My young stomach, new to deprivation, protested with gnawing vigor. Pictures I had seen of famine victims passed wraithlike before me.

"The next Benares death from starvation is due at once in this hermitage," I thought. Impending doom averted at nine o'clock. Ambrosial summons! In memory that meal is vivid as one of life's perfect hours.

Intense absorption yet permitted me to observe that Dyananda ate absent-mindedly. He was apparently above my gross pleasures.

"Swamiji, weren't you hungry?" Happily surfeited, I was alone with the leader in his study.

"O yes! I have spent the last four days without food or drink. I never eat on trains, filled with the heterogenous vibrations of worldly people. Strictly I observe the *shastric*[6] rules for monks of my particular order.

"Certain problems of our organizational work lie on my mind. Tonight at home I neglected my dinner. What's the hurry? Tomorrow I'll make it a point to have a proper meal." He laughed merrily.

Shame spread within me like a suffocation. But the past day of my torture was not easily forgotten; I ventured a further remark.

"Swamiji, I am puzzled. Following your instruction, suppose I never asked for food, and nobody gives me any. I should starve to death."

"Die then!" This alarming counsel split the air. "Die if you must Mukunda! Never admit that you live by the power of food and not by the power of God! He who has created every form of nourishment, He who has bestowed appetite, will certainly see that His devotee is sustained! Do not imagine that rice maintains you, or that money or men support you! Could they aid if the Lord withdraws your life-breath? They are His indirect instruments merely. Is it by any skill of yours that food digests in your stomach? Use the sword of your discrimination, Mukunda! Cut through the chains of agency and perceive the Single Cause!"

I found his incisive words entering some deep marrow. Gone was an age-old delusion by which bodily imperatives outwit the soul. There and then I tasted the Spirit's all-sufficiency. In how many strange cities, in my later life of ceaseless travel, did occasion arise to prove the serviceability of this lesson in a Benares hermitage!

The sole treasure which had accompanied me from Calcutta was the *sadhu's* silver amulet bequeathed to me by Mother. Guarding it for years, I now had it carefully hidden in my ashram room. To renew my joy in the talismanic testimony, one morning I opened the locked box. The sealed covering untouched, lo! the amulet was gone. Mournfully I tore open its envelope and made unmistakably sure. It had vanished, in accordance with the *sadhu's* prediction, into the ether whence he had summoned it.

My relationship with Dyananda's followers grew steadily worse. The household was alienated, hurt by my determined aloofness. My strict adherence to meditation on the very Ideal for which I had left home and all worldly ambitions called forth shallow criticism on all sides.

Torn by spiritual anguish, I entered the attic one dawn, resolved to pray until answer was vouchsafed.

"Merciful Mother of the Universe, teach me Thyself through visions, or through a guru sent by Thee!"

The passing hours found my sobbing pleas without response. Suddenly I felt lifted as though bodily to a sphere uncircumscribed.

"Thy Master cometh today!" A divine womanly voice came from everywhere and nowhere.

This supernal experience was pierced by a shout from a definite locale. A young priest nicknamed Habu was calling me from the downstairs kitchen.

"Mukunda, enough of meditation! You are needed for an errand."

Another day I might have replied impatiently; now I wiped my tear-swollen face and meekly obeyed the summons. Together Habu and I set out for a distant market place in the Bengali section of Benares. The ungentle Indian sun was not yet at zenith as we made our purchases in the bazaars. We pushed our way through the colorful medley of housewives, guides, priests, simply-clad widows, dignified Brahmins, and the ubiquitous holy bulls. Passing an inconspicuous lane, I turned my head and surveyed the narrow length.

A Christlike man in the ocher robes of a swami stood motionless at the end of the road. Instantly and anciently familiar he seemed; my gaze fed hungrily for a trice. Then doubt assailed me.

"You are confusing this wandering monk with someone known to you," I thought. "Dreamer, walk on."

After ten minutes, I felt heavy numbness in my feet. As though turned to stone, they were unable to carry me farther. Laboriously I turned around; my feet regained normalcy. I faced the opposite direction; again the curious weight oppressed me.

"The saint is magnetically drawing me to him!" With this thought, I heaped my parcels into the arms of Habu. He had been observing my erratic footwork with amazement, and now burst into laughter.

"What ails you? Are you crazy?"

My tumultuous emotion prevented any retort; I sped silently away.

Retracing my steps as though wing-shod, I reached the narrow lane. My quick glance revealed the quiet figure, steadily gazing in my direction. A few eager steps and I was at his feet.

"Gurudeva!"[7] The divine face was none other than he of my thousand visions. These halcyon eyes, in leonine head with pointed beard and flowing locks, had oft peered through gloom of my nocturnal reveries, holding a promise I had not fully understood.

"O my own, you have come to me!" My guru uttered the words again and again in Bengali, his voice tremulous with joy. "How many years I have waited for you!"

We entered a oneness of silence; words seemed the rankest superfluities. Eloquence flowed in soundless chant from heart of master to disciple. With an antenna of irrefragable insight I sensed that my guru knew God, and would lead me to Him. The obscuration of this life disappeared in a fragile dawn of prenatal memories. Dramatic time! Past, present, and future are its cycling scenes. This was not the first sun to find me at these holy feet!

My hand in his, my guru led me to his temporary residence in the Rana Mahal section of the city. His athletic figure moved with firm tread. Tall, erect, about fifty-five at this time, he was active and vigorous as a young man. His dark eyes were large, beautiful with plumbless wisdom. Slightly curly hair softened a face of striking power. Strength mingled subtly with gentleness.

As we made our way to the stone balcony of a house overlooking the Ganges, he said affectionately:

"I will give you my hermitages and all I possess."

"Sir, I come for wisdom and God-contact. Those are your treasure-troves I am after!"

The swift Indian twilight had dropped its half-curtain before my master spoke again. His eyes held unfathomable tenderness.

"I give you my unconditional love."

Precious words! A quarter-century elapsed before I had another auricular proof of his love. His lips were strange to ardor; silence became his oceanic heart.

"Will you give me the same unconditional love?" He gazed at me with childlike trust.

"I will love you eternally, Gurudeva!"

"Ordinary love is selfish, darkly rooted in desires and satisfactions. Divine love is without condition, without boundary, without change. The flux of the human heart is gone forever at the transfixing touch of pure love." He added humbly, "If ever you find me falling from a state of God-realization, please promise to put my head on your lap and help to bring me back to the Cosmic Beloved we both worship."

He rose then in the gathering darkness and guided me to an inner room. As we ate mangoes and almond sweetmeats, he unobtrusively wove into his conversation an intimate knowledge of my nature. I was awe-struck at the grandeur of his wisdom, exquisitely blended with an innate humility.

"Do not grieve for your amulet. It has served its purpose." Like a divine mirror, my guru apparently had caught a reflection of my whole life.

"The living reality of your presence, Master, is joy beyond any symbol."

"It is time for a change, inasmuch as you are unhappily situated in the hermitage."

I had made no references to my life; they now seemed superfluous! By his natural, unemphatic manner, I understood that he wished no astonished ejaculations at his clairvoyance.

"You should go back to Calcutta. Why exclude relatives from your love of humanity?"

His suggestion dismayed me. My family was predicting my return, though I had been unresponsive to many pleas by letter. "Let the young bird fly in the metaphysical skies," Ananta had remarked. "His wings will tire in the heavy atmosphere. We shall yet see him swoop toward home, fold his pinions, and humbly rest in our family nest." This discouraging simile fresh in my mind, I was determined to do no "swooping" in the direction of Calcutta.

"Sir, I am not returning home. But I will follow you anywhere. Please give me your address, and your name."

"Swami Sri Yukteswar Giri. My chief hermitage is in Serampore, on Rai Ghat Lane. I am visiting my mother here for only a few days."

I wondered at God's intricate play with His devotees. Serampore is but twelve miles from Calcutta, yet in those regions I had never caught a glimpse of my guru. We had had to travel for our meeting to the ancient city of Kasi (Benares), hallowed by memories of Lahiri Mahasaya. Here too the feet of Buddha, Shankaracharya and other Yogi-Christs had blessed the soil.

"You will come to me in four weeks." For the first time, Sri Yukteswar's voice was stern. "Now I have told my eternal affection, and have shown my happiness at finding you-that is why you disregard my request. The next time we meet, you will have to reawaken my interest: I won't accept you as a disciple easily. There must be complete surrender by obedience to my strict training."

I remained obstinately silent. My guru easily penetrated my difficulty.

"Do you think your relatives will laugh at you?"

"I will not return."

"You will return in thirty days."

"Never." Bowing reverently at his feet, I departed without lightening the controversial tension. As I made my way in the midnight darkness, I wondered why the miraculous meeting had ended on an inharmonious note. The dual scales of *maya,* that balance every joy with a grief! My young heart was not yet malleable to the transforming fingers of my guru.

The next morning I noticed increased hostility in the attitude of the hermitage members. My days became spiked with invariable rudeness. In three weeks, Dyananda left the ashram to attend a conference in Bombay; pandemonium broke over my hapless head.

"Mukunda is a parasite, accepting hermitage hospitality without making proper return." Overhearing this remark, I regretted for the first time that I had obeyed the request to send back my money to Father. With heavy heart, I sought out my sole friend, Jitendra.

"I am leaving. Please convey my respectful regrets to Dyanandaji when he returns."

"I will leave also! My attempts to meditate here meet with no more favor than your own." Jitendra spoke with determination.

"I have met a Christlike saint. Let us visit him in Serampore."

And so the "bird" prepared to "swoop" perilously close to Calcutta!

---

[1] Sanskrita, polished; complete. Sanskrit is the eldest sister of all Indo-European tongues. Its alphabetical script is Devanagari, literally "divine abode." "Who knows my grammar knows God!" Panini, great philologist of ancient India, paid this tribute to the mathematical and psychological perfection in Sanskrit. He who would track language to its lair must indeed end as omniscient.

[2] He was not Jatinda (Jotin Ghosh), who will be remembered for his timely aversion to tigers!

[3] Path or preliminary road to God.

[4] Hindu scriptures teach that family attachment is delusive if it prevents the devotee from seeking the Giver of all boons, including the one of loving relatives, not to mention life itself. Jesus similarly taught: "Who is my mother? and who are my brethren?" (Matthew 12:48.)

[5] Ji is a customary respectful suffix, particularly used in direct address; thus "swamiji," "guruji," "Sri Yukteswarji," "paramhansaji."

[6] Pertaining to the shastras, literally, "sacred books," comprising four classes of scripture: the shruti, smriti, purana, and tantra. These comprehensive treatises cover every aspect of religious and social life, and the fields of law, medicine, architecture, art, etc. The shrutis are the "directly heard" or "revealed" scriptures, the Vedas. The smritis or "remembered" lore was finally written down in a remote past as the world's longest epic poems, the Mahabharata and the Ramayana. Puranas are literally "ancient" allegories; tantras literally mean "rites" or "rituals"; these treatises convey profound truths under a veil of detailed symbolism.

[7] "Divine teacher," the customary Sanskrit term for one's spiritual preceptor. I have rendered it in English as simply "Master."

## CHAPTER 12

# *Years in My Master's Hermitage*

"You have come." Sri Yukteswar greeted me from a tiger skin on the floor of a balconied sitting room. His voice was cold, his manner unemotional.

"Yes, dear Master, I am here to follow you." Kneeling, I touched his feet.

"How can that be? You ignore my wishes."

"No longer, Guruji! Your wish shall be my law!"

"That is better! Now I can assume responsibility for your life."

"I willingly transfer the burden, Master."

"My first request, then, is that you return home to your family. I want you to enter college in Calcutta. Your education should be continued."

"Very well, sir." I hid my consternation. Would importunate books pursue me down the years? First Father, now Sri Yukteswar!

"Someday you will go to the West. Its people will lend ears more receptive to India's ancient wisdom if the strange Hindu teacher has a university degree."

"You know best, Guruji." My gloom departed. The reference to the West I found puzzling, remote; but my opportunity to please Master by obedience was vitally immediate.

"You will be near in Calcutta; come here whenever you find time."

"Every day if possible, Master! Gratefully I accept your authority in every detail of my life-on one condition."

"Yes?"

"That you promise to reveal God to me!"

An hour-long verbal tussle ensued. A master's word cannot be falsified; it is not lightly given. The implications in the pledge open out vast metaphysical vistas. A guru must be on intimate terms indeed with the Creator before he can obligate Him to appear! I sensed Sri Yukteswar's divine unity, and was determined, as his disciple, to press my advantage.

"You are of exacting disposition!" Then Master's consent rang out with compassionate finality:

"Let your wish be my wish."

Lifelong shadow lifted from my heart; the vague search, hither and yon, was over. I had found eternal shelter in a true guru.

"Come; I will show you the hermitage." Master rose from his tiger mat. I glanced about me; my gaze fell with astonishment on a wall picture, garlanded with a spray of jasmine.

"Lahiri Mahasaya!"

"Yes, my divine guru." Sri Yukteswar's tone was reverently vibrant. "Greater he was, as man and yogi, than any other teacher whose life came within the range of my investigations."

Silently I bowed before the familiar picture. Soul-homage sped to the peerless master who, blessing my infancy, had guided my steps to this hour.

Led by my guru, I strolled over the house and its grounds. Large, ancient and well-built, the hermitage was surrounded by a massive-pillared courtyard. Outer walls were moss-covered; pigeons fluttered over the flat gray roof, unceremoniously sharing the ashram quarters. A rear garden was pleasant with jackfruit, mango, and plantain trees. Balustraded balconies of upper rooms in the two-storied building faced the courtyard from three sides. A spacious ground-floor hall, with high ceiling supported by colonnades, was used, Master said, chiefly during the annual festivities of *Durgapuja*.[1] A narrow stairway led to Sri Yukteswar's sitting room, whose small balcony overlooked the street. The ashram was plainly furnished; everything was simple, clean, and utilitarian. Several Western styled chairs, benches, and tables were in evidence.

Master invited me to stay overnight. A supper of vegetable curry was served by two young disciples who were receiving hermitage training.

"Guruji, please tell me something of your life." I was squatting on a straw mat near his tiger skin. The friendly stars were very close, it seemed, beyond the balcony.

"My family name was Priya Nath Karar. I was born[2] here in Serampore, where Father was a wealthy businessman. He left me this ancestral mansion, now my hermitage. My formal schooling was little; I found it slow and shallow. In early manhood, I undertook the responsibilities of a householder, and have one daughter, now married. My middle life was blessed with the guidance of Lahiri Mahasaya. After my wife died, I joined the Swami Order and received the new name of Sri Yukteswar Giri.[3] Such are my simple annals."

Master smiled at my eager face. Like all biographical sketches, his words had given the outward facts without revealing the inner man.

"Guruji, I would like to hear some stories of your childhood."

"I will tell you a few-each one with a moral!" Sri Yukteswar's eyes twinkled with his warning. "My mother once tried to frighten me with an appalling story of a ghost in a dark chamber. I went there immediately, and expressed my disappointment at having missed the ghost. Mother never told me another horror-tale. Moral: Look fear in the face and it will cease to trouble you.

"Another early memory is my wish for an ugly dog belonging to a neighbor. I kept my household in turmoil for weeks to get that dog. My ears were deaf to offers of pets with more prepossessing appearance. Moral: Attachment is blinding; it lends an imaginary halo of attractiveness to the object of desire.

"A third story concerns the plasticity of the youthful mind. I heard my mother remark occasionally: 'A man who accepts a job under anyone is a slave.' That impression became so indelibly fixed that even after my marriage I refused all positions. I met expenses by investing my family endowment in land. Moral: Good and positive suggestions should instruct the sensitive ears of children. Their early ideas long remain sharply etched."

Master fell into tranquil silence. Around midnight he led me to a narrow cot. Sleep was sound and sweet the first night under my guru's roof.

Sri Yukteswar chose the following morning to grant me his *Kriya Yoga* initiation. The technique I had already received from two disciples of Lahiri Mahasaya - Father and my tutor, Swami Kebalananda - but in Master's presence I felt transforming power. At his touch, a great light broke upon my being, like glory of countless suns blazing together. A flood of ineffable bliss, overwhelming my heart to an innermost core, continued during the following day. It was late that afternoon before I could bring myself to leave the hermitage.

"You will return in thirty days." As I reached my Calcutta home, the fulfillment of Master's prediction entered with me. None of my relatives made the pointed remarks I had feared about the reappearance of the "soaring bird."

I climbed to my little attic and bestowed affectionate glances, as though on a living presence. "You have witnessed my meditations, and the tears and storms of my *sadhana.* Now I have reached the harbor of my divine teacher."

"Son, I am happy for us both." Father and I sat together in the evening calm. "You have found your guru, as in miraculous fashion I once found my own. The holy hand of Lahiri Mahasaya is guarding our lives. Your master has proved no inaccessible Himalayan saint, but one near-by. My prayers have been answered: you have not in your search for God been permanently removed from my sight."

Father was also pleased that my formal studies would be resumed; he made suitable arrangements. I was enrolled the following day at the Scottish Church College in Calcutta.

Happy months sped by. My readers have doubtless made the perspicacious surmise that I was little seen in the college classrooms. The Serampore hermitage held a lure too irresistible. Master accepted my ubiquitous presence without comment. To my relief, he seldom referred to the halls of learning. Though it was plain to all that I was never cut out for a scholar, I managed to attain minimum passing grades from time to time.

Daily life at the ashram flowed smoothly, infrequently varied. My guru awoke before dawn. Lying down, or sometimes sitting on the bed, he entered a state of *samadh.*[4] It was simplicity itself to discover when Master had awakened: abrupt halt of stupendous snores.[5] A sigh or two; perhaps a bodily movement. Then a soundless state of breathlessness: he was in deep yogic joy.

Breakfast did not follow; first came a long walk by the Ganges. Those morning strolls with my guru-how real and vivid still! In the easy resurrection of memory, I often find myself by his side: the early sun is warming the river. His voice rings out, rich with the authenticity of wisdom.

A bath; then the midday meal. Its preparation, according to Master's daily directions, had been the careful task of young disciples. My guru was a vegetarian. Before embracing monkhood, however, he had eaten eggs and fish. His advice to students was to follow any simple diet which proved suited to one's constitution.

Master ate little; often rice, colored with turmeric or juice of beets or spinach and lightly sprinkled with buffalo *ghee* or melted butter. Another day he might have lentil-*dhal* or *channa*[6] - curry with vegetables. For dessert, mangoes or oranges with rice pudding, or jackfruit juice.

Visitors appeared in the afternoons. A steady stream poured from the world into the hermitage tranquillity. Everyone found in Master an equal courtesy and kindness. To a man who has realized himself as a soul, not the body or the ego, the rest of humanity assumes a striking similarity of aspect.

The impartiality of saints is rooted in wisdom. Masters have escaped *maya;* its alternating faces of intellect and idiocy no longer cast an influential glance. Sri Yukteswar showed no special consideration to those who happened to be powerful or accomplished; neither did he slight others for their poverty or illiteracy. He would listen respectfully to words of truth from a child, and openly ignore a conceited pundit.

Eight o'clock was the supper hour, and sometimes found lingering guests. My guru would not excuse himself to eat alone; none left his ashram hungry or dissatisfied. Sri Yukteswar was never at a loss, never dismayed by unexpected visitors; scanty food would emerge a banquet under his resourceful direction. Yet he was economical; his modest funds went far. "Be comfortable within your purse," he often said. "Extravagance will buy you discomfort." Whether in the details of hermitage entertainment, or his building and repair work, or other practical concerns, Master manifested the originality of a creative spirit.

Quiet evening hours often brought one of my guru's discourses, treasures against time. His every utterance was measured and chiseled by wisdom. A sublime self-assurance marked his mode of expression: it was unique. He spoke as none other in my experience ever spoke. His thoughts were weighed in a delicate balance of discrimination before he permitted them an outward garb. The essence of truth, all-pervasive with even a physiological aspect, came from him like a fragrant exudation of the soul. I was conscious always that I was in the presence of a living manifestation of God. The weight of his divinity automatically bowed my head before him.

If late guests detected that Sri Yukteswar was becoming engrossed with the Infinite, he quickly engaged them in conversation. He was incapable of striking a pose, or of flaunting his inner withdrawal. Always one with the Lord, he needed no separate time for communion. A self-realized master has already left behind the stepping stone of meditation. "The flower falls when the fruit appears." But saints often cling to spiritual forms for the encouragement of disciples.

As midnight approached, my guru might fall into a doze with the naturalness of a child. There was no fuss about bedding. He often lay down, without even a pillow, on a narrow davenport which was the background for his customary tiger-skin seat.

A night-long philosophical discussion was not rare; any disciple could summon it by intensity of interest. I felt no tiredness then, no desire for sleep; Master's living words were sufficient. "Oh, it is dawn! Let us walk by the Ganges." So ended many of my periods of nocturnal edification.

My early months with Sri Yukteswar culminated in a useful lesson-"How to Outwit a Mosquito." At home my family always used protective curtains at night. I was dismayed to discover that in the Serampore hermitage this prudent custom was honored in the breach. Yet the insects were in full residency; I was bitten from head to foot. My guru took pity on me.

"Buy yourself a curtain, and also one for me." He laughed and added, "If you buy only one, for yourself, all mosquitoes will concentrate on me!"

I was more than thankful to comply. Every night that I spent in Serampore, my guru would ask me to arrange the bedtime curtains.

The mosquitoes one evening were especially virulent. But Master failed to issue his usual instructions. I listened nervously to the anticipatory hum of the insects. Getting into bed, I threw a propitiatory prayer in their general direction. A half hour later, I coughed pretentiously to attract my guru's attention. I thought I would go mad with the bites and especially the singing drone as the mosquitoes celebrated bloodthirsty rites.

No responsive stir from Master; I approached him cautiously. He was not breathing. This was my first observation of him in the yogic trance; it filled me with fright.

"His heart must have failed!" I placed a mirror under his nose; no breath-vapor appeared. To make doubly certain, for minutes I closed his mouth and nostrils with my fingers. His body was cold and motionless. In a daze, I turned toward the door to summon help.

"So! A budding experimentalist! My poor nose!" Master's voice was shaky with laughter. "Why don't you go to bed? Is the whole world going to change for you? Change yourself: be rid of the mosquito consciousness."

Meekly I returned to my bed. Not one insect ventured near. I realized that my guru had previously agreed to the curtains only to please me; he had no fear of mosquitoes. His yogic power was such that he either could will them not to bite, or could escape to an inner invulnerability.

"He was giving me a demonstration," I thought. "That is the yogic state I must strive to attain." A yogi must be able to pass into, and continue in, the superconsciousness, regardless of multitudinous distractions never absent from this earth. Whether in the buzz of insects or the pervasive glare of daylight, the testimony of the senses must be barred. Sound and sight come then indeed, but to worlds fairer than the banished Eden.[7]

The instructive mosquitoes served for another early lesson at the ashram. It was the gentle hour of dusk. My guru was matchlessly interpreting the ancient texts. At his feet, I was in perfect peace. A rude mosquito entered the idyll and competed for my attention. As it dug a poisonous hypodermic needle into my thigh, I automatically raised an avenging hand. Reprieve from impending execution! An opportune memory came to me of one of Patanjali's yoga aphorisms - that on *ahimsa* (harmlessness).

"Why didn't you finish the job?"

"Master! Do you advocate taking life?"

"No; but the deathblow already had been struck in your mind."

"I don't understand."

"Patanjali's meaning was the removal of *desire* to kill." Sri Yukteswar had found my mental processes an open book. "This world is inconveniently arranged for a literal practice of *ahimsa.* Man may be compelled to exterminate harmful creatures. He is not under similar compulsion to feel anger or animosity. All forms of life have equal right to the air of *maya.* The saint who uncovers the secret of creation will be in harmony with its countless bewildering expressions. All men may approach that understanding who curb the inner passion for destruction."

"Guruji, should one offer himself a sacrifice rather than kill a wild beast?"

"No; man's body is precious. It has the highest evolutionary value because of unique brain and spinal centers. These enable the advanced devotee to fully grasp and express the loftiest aspects of divinity. No lower form is so equipped. It is true that one incurs the debt of a minor sin if he is forced to kill an animal or any living thing. But the *Vedas* teach that wanton loss of a human body is a serious transgression against the karmic law."

I sighed in relief; scriptural reinforcement of one's natural instincts is not always forthcoming.

It so happened that I never saw Master at close quarters with a leopard or a tiger. But a deadly cobra once confronted him, only to be conquered by my guru's love. This variety of snake is much feared in India, where it causes more than five thousand deaths annually. The dangerous encounter took place at Puri, where Sri Yukteswar had a second hermitage, charmingly situated near the Bay of Bengal. Prafulla, a young disciple of later years, was with Master on this occasion.

"We were seated outdoors near the ashram," Prafulla told me. "A cobra appeared near-by, a four-foot length of sheer terror. Its hood was angrily expanded as it raced toward us. My guru gave a welcoming chuckle, as though to a child. I was beside myself with consternation to see Master engage in a rhythmical clapping of hands.[8] He was entertaining the dread visitor! I remained absolutely quiet, inwardly ejaculating what fervent prayers I could muster. The serpent, very close to my guru, was now motionless, seemingly magnetized by his caressing attitude. The frightful hood gradually contracted; the snake slithered between Master's feet and disappeared into the bushes.

"Why my guru would move his hands, and why the cobra would not strike them, were inexplicable to me then," Prafulla concluded. "I have since come to realize that my divine master is beyond fear of hurt from any living creature."

One afternoon during my early months at the ashram, found Sri Yukteswar's eyes fixed on me piercingly.

"You are too thin, Mukunda."

His remark struck a sensitive point. That my sunken eyes and emaciated appearance were far from my liking was testified to by rows of tonics in my room at Calcutta. Nothing availed; chronic dyspepsia had pursued me since childhood. My despair reached an occasional zenith when I asked myself if it were worth-while to carry on this life with a body so unsound.

"Medicines have limitations; the creative life-force has none. Believe that: you shall be well and strong."

Sri Yukteswar's words aroused a conviction of personally-applicable truth which no other healer-and I had tried many!-had been able to summon within me.

Day by day, behold! I waxed. Two weeks after Master's hidden blessing, I had accumulated the invigorating weight which eluded me in the past. My persistent stomach ailments vanished with a lifelong permanency. On later occasions I witnessed my guru's instantaneous divine healings of persons suffering from ominous disease-tuberculosis, diabetes, epilepsy, or paralysis. Not one could have been more grateful for his cure than I was at sudden freedom from my cadaverous aspect.

"Years ago, I too was anxious to put on weight," Sri Yukteswar told me. "During convalescence after a severe illness, I visited Lahiri Mahasaya in Benares.

"Sir, I have been very sick and lost many pounds."

"I see, Yukteswar,[9] you made yourself unwell, and now you think you are thin."

"This reply was far from the one I had expected; my guru, however, added encouragingly:

"Let me see; I am sure you ought to feel better tomorrow."

"Taking his words as a gesture of secret healing toward my receptive mind, I was not surprised the next morning at a welcome accession of strength. I sought out my master and exclaimed exultingly, 'Sir, I feel much better today.'

"Indeed! Today you invigorate yourself.'

"No, master!' I protested. 'It was you who helped me; this is the first time in weeks that I have had any energy.'

"O yes! Your malady has been quite serious. Your body is frail yet; who can say how it will be tomorrow?'

"The thought of possible return of my weakness brought me a shudder of cold fear. The following morning I could hardly drag myself to Lahiri Mahasaya's home.

"Sir, I am ailing again.'

"My guru's glance was quizzical. 'So! Once more you indispose yourself.'

"Gurudeva, I realize now that day by day you have been ridiculing me.' My patience was exhausted. 'I don't understand why you disbelieve my truthful reports.'

"Really, it has been your thoughts that have made you feel alternately weak and strong.' My master looked at me affectionately. 'You have seen how your health has exactly followed your expectations. Thought is a force, even as electricity or gravitation. The human mind is a spark of the almighty consciousness of God. I could show you that whatever your powerful mind believes very intensely would instantly come to pass.'

"Knowing that Lahiri Mahasaya never spoke idly, I addressed him with great awe and gratitude: 'Master, if I think I am well and have regained my former weight, shall that happen?'

"It is so, even at this moment.' My guru spoke gravely, his gaze concentrated on my eyes.

"Lo! I felt an increase not alone of strength but of weight. Lahiri Mahasaya retreated into silence. After a few hours at his feet, I returned to my mother's home, where I stayed during my visits to Benares.

"My son! What is the matter? Are you swelling with dropsy?' Mother could hardly believe her eyes. My body was now of the same robust dimensions it had possessed before my illness.

"I weighed myself and found that in one day I had gained fifty pounds; they remained with me permanently. Friends and acquaintances who had seen my thin figure were aghast with wonderment. A number of them changed their mode of life and became disciples of Lahiri Mahasaya as a result of this miracle.

"My guru, awake in God, knew this world to be nothing but an objectivized dream of the Creator. Because he was completely aware of his unity with the Divine Dreamer, Lahiri Mahasaya could materialize or dematerialize or make any change he wished in the cosmic vision.[10]

"All creation is governed by law," Sri Yukteswar concluded. "The ones which manifest in the outer universe, discoverable by scientists, are called natural laws. But there are subtler laws ruling the realms of consciousness which can be known only through the inner science of yoga. The hidden spiritual planes also have their natural and lawful principles of operation. It is not the physical scientist but the fully self-realized master who comprehends the true nature of matter. Thus Christ was able to restore the servant's ear after it had been severed by one of the disciples."[11]

Sri Yukteswar was a peerless interpreter of the scriptures. Many of my happiest memories are centered in his discourses. But his jeweled thoughts were not cast into ashes of heedlessness or stupidity. One restless movement of my body, or my slight lapse into absent-mindedness, sufficed to put an abrupt period to Master's exposition.

"You are not here." Master interrupted himself one afternoon with this disclosure. As usual, he was keeping track of my attention with a devastating immediacy.

"Guruji!" My tone was a protest. "I have not stirred; my eyelids have not moved; I can repeat each word you have uttered!"

"Nevertheless you were not fully with me. Your objection forces me to remark that in your mental background you were creating three institutions. One was a sylvan retreat on a plain, another on a hilltop, a third by the ocean."

Those vaguely formulated thoughts had indeed been present almost subconsciously. I glanced at him apologetically.

"What can I do with such a master, who penetrates my random musings?"

"You have given me that right. The subtle truths I am expounding cannot be grasped without your complete concentration. Unless necessary I do not invade the seclusion of others' minds. Man has the natural privilege of roaming secretly among his thoughts. The unbidden Lord does not enter there; neither do I venture intrusion."

"You are ever welcome, Master!"

"Your architectural dreams will materialize later. Now is the time for study!"

Thus incidentally my guru revealed in his simple way the coming of three great events in my life. Since early youth I had had enigmatic glimpses of three buildings, each in a different setting. In the exact sequence Sri Yukteswar had indicated, these visions took ultimate form. First came my founding of a boys' yoga school on a Ranchi plain, then my American headquarters on a Los Angeles hilltop, finally a hermitage in southern California by the vast Pacific.

Master never arrogantly asserted: "I prophesy that such and such an event shall occur!" He would rather hint: "Don't you think it may happen?" But his simple speech hid vatic power. There was no recanting; never did his slightly veiled words prove false.

Sri Yukteswar was reserved and matter-of-fact in demeanor. There was naught of the vague or daft visionary about him. His feet were firm on the earth, his head in the haven of heaven. Practical people aroused his admiration. "Saintliness is not dumbness! Divine perceptions are not incapacitating!" he would say. "The active expression of virtue gives rise to the keenest intelligence."

In Master's life I fully discovered the cleavage between spiritual realism and the obscure mysticism that spuriously passes as a counterpart. My guru was reluctant to discuss the superphysical realms. His only "marvelous" aura was one of perfect simplicity. In conversation he avoided startling references; in action he was freely expressive. Others talked of miracles but could manifest nothing; Sri Yukteswar seldom mentioned the subtle laws but secretly operated them at will.

"A man of realization does not perform any miracle until he receives an inward sanction," Master explained. "God does not wish the secrets of His creation revealed promiscuously.[12] Also, every individual in the world has inalienable right to his free will. A saint will not encroach upon that independence."

The silence habitual to Sri Yukteswar was caused by his deep perceptions of the Infinite. No time remained for the interminable "revelations" that occupy the days of teachers without self-realization. "In shallow men the fish of little thoughts cause much commotion. In oceanic minds the whales of inspiration make hardly a ruffle." This observation from the Hindu scriptures is not without discerning humor.

Because of my guru's unspectacular guise, only a few of his contemporaries recognized him as a superman. The popular adage: "He is a fool that cannot conceal his wisdom," could never be applied to Sri Yukteswar. Though born a mortal like all others, Master had achieved identity with the Ruler of time and space. In his life I perceived a godlike unity. He had not found any insuperable obstacle to mergence of human with Divine. No such barrier exists, I came to understand, save in man's spiritual unadventurousness.

I always thrilled at the touch of Sri Yukteswar's holy feet. Yogis teach that a disciple is spiritually magnetized by reverent contact with a master; a subtle current is generated. The devotee's undesirable habit-mechanisms in the brain are often cauterized; the groove of his worldly tendencies beneficially disturbed.

Momentarily at least he may find the secret veils of *maya* lifting, and glimpse the reality of bliss. My whole body responded with a liberating glow whenever I knelt in the Indian fashion before my guru.

"Even when Lahiri Mahasaya was silent," Master told me, "or when he conversed on other than strictly religious topics, I discovered that nonetheless he had transmitted to me ineffable knowledge."

Sri Yukteswar affected me similarly. If I entered the hermitage in a worried or indifferent frame of mind, my attitude imperceptibly changed. A healing calm descended at mere sight of my guru. Every day with him was a new experience in joy, peace, and wisdom. Never did I find him deluded or intoxicated with greed or emotion or anger or any human attachment.

"The darkness of *maya* is silently approaching. Let us hie homeward within." With these words at dusk Master constantly reminded his disciples of their need for *Kriya Yoga.* A new student occasionally expressed doubts regarding his own worthiness to engage in yoga practice.

"Forget the past," Sri Yukteswar would console him. "The vanished lives of all men are dark with many shames. Human conduct is ever unreliable until anchored in the Divine. Everything in future will improve if you are making a spiritual effort now."

Master always had young *chelas*[13] in his hermitage. Their spiritual and intellectual education was his lifelong interest: even shortly before he passed on, he accepted for training two six-year-old boys and one youth of sixteen. He directed their minds and lives with that careful discipline in which the word "disciple" is etymologically rooted. The ashram residents loved and revered their guru; a slight clap of his hands sufficed to bring them eagerly to his side. When his mood was silent and withdrawn, no one ventured to speak; when his laugh rang jovially, children looked upon him as their own.

Master seldom asked others to render him a personal service, nor would he accept help from a student unless the willingness were sincere. My guru quietly washed his clothes if the disciples overlooked that privileged task. Sri Yukteswar wore the traditional ocher-colored swami robe; his laceless shoes, in accordance with yogi custom, were of tiger or deer skin.

Master spoke fluent English, French, Hindi, and Bengali; his Sanskrit was fair. He patiently instructed his young disciples by certain short cuts which he had ingeniously devised for the study of English and Sanskrit.

Master was cautious of his body, while withholding solicitous attachment. The Infinite, he pointed out, properly manifests through physical and mental soundness. He discountenanced any extremes. A disciple once started a long fast. My guru only laughed: "Why not throw the dog a bone?"

Sri Yukteswar's health was excellent; I never saw him unwell.[14] He permitted students to consult doctors if it seemed advisable. His purpose was to give respect to the worldly custom: "Physicians must carry on their work of healing through God's laws as applied to matter." But he extolled the superiority of mental therapy, and often repeated: "Wisdom is the greatest cleanser."

"The body is a treacherous friend. Give it its due; no more," he said. "Pain and pleasure are transitory; endure all dualities with calmness, while trying at the same time to remove their hold. Imagination is the door through which disease as well as healing enters. Disbelieve in the reality of sickness even when you are ill; an unrecognized visitor will flee!"

Master numbered many doctors among his disciples. "Those who have ferreted out the physical laws can easily investigate the science of the soul," he told them. "A subtle spiritual mechanism is hidden just behind the bodily structure."[15]

Sri Yukteswar counseled his students to be living liaisons of Western and Eastern virtues. Himself an executive Occidental in outer habits, inwardly he was the spiritual Oriental. He praised the progressive, resourceful and hygienic habits of the West, and the religious ideals which give a centuried halo to the East.

Discipline had not been unknown to me: at home Father was strict, Ananta often severe. But Sri Yukteswar's training cannot be described as other than drastic. A perfectionist, my guru was hypercritical of his disciples, whether in matters of moment or in the subtle nuances of behavior.

"Good manners without sincerity are like a beautiful dead lady," he remarked on suitable occasion. "Straightforwardness without civility is like a surgeon's knife, effective but unpleasant. Candor with courtesy is helpful and admirable."

Master was apparently satisfied with my spiritual progress, for he seldom referred to it; in other matters my ears were no strangers to reproof. My chief offenses were absentmindedness, intermittent indulgence in sad moods, non-observance of certain rules of etiquette, and occasional unmethodical ways.

"Observe how the activities of your father Bhagabati are well-organized and balanced in every way," my guru pointed out. The two disciples of Lahiri Mahasaya had met, soon after I began my pilgrimages to Serampore. Father and Sri Yukteswar admiringly evaluated the other's worth. Both had built an inner life of spiritual granite, insoluble against the ages.

From transient teachers of my earlier life I had imbibed a few erroneous lessons. A *chela*, I was told, need not concern himself strenuously over worldly duties; when I had neglected or carelessly performed my tasks, I was not chastised. Human nature finds such instruction very easy of assimilation. Under Master's unsparing rod, however, I soon recovered from the agreeable delusions of irresponsibility.

"Those who are too good for this world are adorning some other," Sri Yukteswar remarked. "So long as you breathe the free air of earth, you are under obligation to render grateful service. He alone who has fully mastered the breathless state[16] is freed from cosmic imperatives. I will not fail to let you know when you have attained the final perfection."

My guru could never be bribed, even by love. He showed no leniency to anyone who, like myself, willingly offered to be his disciple. Whether Master and I were surrounded by his students or by strangers, or were alone together, he always spoke plainly and upbraided sharply. No trifling lapse into shallowness or inconsistency escaped his rebuke. This flattening treatment was hard to endure, but my resolve was to allow Sri Yukteswar to iron out each of my psychological kinks. As he labored at this titanic transformation, I shook many times under the weight of his disciplinary hammer.

"If you don't like my words, you are at liberty to leave at any time," Master assured me. "I want nothing from you but your own improvement. Stay only if you feel benefited."

For every humbling blow he dealt my vanity, for every tooth in my metaphorical jaw he knocked loose with stunning aim, I am grateful beyond any facility of expression. The hard core of human egotism is hardly to be dislodged except rudely. With its departure, the Divine finds at last an unobstructed channel. In vain It seeks to percolate through flinty hearts of selfishness.

Sri Yukteswar's wisdom was so penetrating that, heedless of remarks, he often replied to one's unspoken observation. "What a person imagines he hears, and what the speaker has really implied, may be poles apart," he said. "Try to feel the thoughts behind the confusion of men's verbiage."

But divine insight is painful to worldly ears; Master was not popular with superficial students. The wise, always few in number, deeply revered him. I daresay Sri Yukteswar would have been the most sought-after guru in India had his words not been so candid and so censorious.

"I am hard on those who come for my training," he admitted to me. "That is my way; take it or leave it. I will never compromise. But you will be much kinder to your disciples; that is your way. I try to purify only in the fires of severity, searing beyond the average toleration. The gentle approach of love is also transfiguring. The inflexible and the yielding methods are equally effective if applied with wisdom. You will go to foreign lands, where blunt assaults on the ego are not appreciated. A teacher could not spread India's message in the West without an ample fund of accommodative patience and forbearance." I refuse to state the amount of truth I later came to find in Master's words!

Though Sri Yukteswar's undissembling speech prevented a large following during his years on earth, nevertheless his living spirit manifests today over the world, through sincere students of his *Kriya Yoga* and other teachings. He has further dominion in men's souls than ever Alexander dreamed of in the soil.

Father arrived one day to pay his respects to Sri Yukteswar. My parent expected, very likely, to hear some words in my praise. He was shocked to be given a long account of my imperfections. It was Master's practice to recount simple, negligible shortcomings with an air of portentous gravity. Father rushed to see me. "From your guru's remarks I thought to find you a complete wreck!" My parent was between tears and laughter.

The only cause of Sri Yukteswar's displeasure at the time was that I had been trying, against his gentle hint, to convert a certain man to the spiritual path.

With indignant speed I sought out my guru. He received me with downcast eyes, as though conscious of guilt. It was the only time I ever saw the divine lion meek before me. The unique moment was savored to the full.

"Sir, why did you judge me so mercilessly before my astounded father? Was that just?"

"I will not do it again." Master's tone was apologetic.

Instantly I was disarmed. How readily the great man admitted his fault! Though he never again upset Father's peace of mind, Master relentlessly continued to dissect me whenever and wherever he chose.

New disciples often joined Sri Yukteswar in exhaustive criticism of others. Wise like the guru! Models of flawless discrimination! But he who takes the offensive must not be defenseless. The same carping students fled precipitantly as soon as Master publicly unloosed in their direction a few shafts from his analytical quiver.

"Tender inner weaknesses, revolting at mild touches of censure, are like diseased parts of the body, recoiling before even delicate handling." This was Sri Yukteswar's amused comment on the flighty ones.

There are disciples who seek a guru made in their own image. Such students often complained that they did not understand Sri Yukteswar.

"Neither do you comprehend God!" I retorted on one occasion. "When a saint is clear to you, you will be one." Among the trillion mysteries, breathing every second the inexplicable air, who may venture to ask that the fathomless nature of a master be instantly grasped?

Students came, and generally went. Those who craved a path of oily sympathy and comfortable recognitions did not find it at the hermitage. Master offered shelter and shepherding for the aeons, but many disciples miserly demanded ego-balm as well. They departed, preferring life's countless humiliations before any humility. Master's blazing rays, the open penetrating sunshine of his wisdom, were too powerful for their spiritual sickness. They sought some lesser teacher who, shading them with flattery, permitted the fitful sleep of ignorance.

During my early months with Master, I had experienced a sensitive fear of his reprimands. These were reserved, I soon saw, for disciples who had asked for his verbal vivisection. If any writhing student made a protest, Sri Yukteswar would become unoffendedly silent. His words were never wrathful, but impersonal with wisdom.

Master's insight was not for the unprepared ears of casual visitors; he seldom remarked on their defects, even if conspicuous. But toward students who sought his counsel, Sri Yukteswar felt a serious responsibility. Brave indeed is the guru who undertakes to transform the crude ore of ego-permeated humanity! A saint's courage roots in his compassion for the stumbling eyeless of this world.

When I had abandoned underlying resentment, I found a marked decrease in my chastisement. In a very subtle way, Master melted into comparative clemency. In time I demolished every wall of rationalization and subconscious reservation behind which the human personality generally shields itself.[17] The reward was an effortless harmony with my guru. I discovered him then to be trusting, considerate, and silently loving. Undemonstrative, however, he bestowed no word of affection.

My own temperament is principally devotional. It was disconcerting at first to find that my guru, saturated with *jnana* but seemingly dry of *bhakti*,[18] expressed himself only in terms of cold spiritual mathematics. But as I tuned myself to his nature, I discovered no diminution but rather increase in my devotional approach to God. A self-realized master is fully able to guide his various disciples along natural lines of their essential bias.

My relationship with Sri Yukteswar, somewhat inarticulate, nonetheless possessed all eloquence. Often I found his silent signature on my thoughts, rendering speech inutile. Quietly sitting beside him, I felt his bounty pouring peacefully over my being.

Sri Yukteswar's impartial justice was notably demonstrated during the summer vacation of my first college year. I welcomed the opportunity to spend uninterrupted months at Serampore with my guru.

"You may be in charge of the hermitage." Master was pleased over my enthusiastic arrival. "Your duties will be the reception of guests, and supervision of the work of the other disciples."

Kumar, a young villager from east Bengal, was accepted a fortnight later for hermitage training. Remarkably intelligent, he quickly won Sri Yukteswar's affection. For some unfathomable reason, Master was very lenient to the new resident.

"Mukunda, let Kumar assume your duties. Employ your own time in sweeping and cooking." Master issued these instructions after the new boy had been with us for a month.

Exalted to leadership, Kumar exercised a petty household tyranny. In silent mutiny, the other disciples continued to seek me out for daily counsel.

"Mukunda is impossible! You made me supervisor, yet the others go to him and obey him." Three weeks later Kumar was complaining to our guru. I overheard him from an adjoining room.

"That's why I assigned him to the kitchen and you to the parlor." Sri Yukteswar's withering tones were new to Kumar. "In this way you have come to realize that a worthy leader has the desire to serve, and not to dominate. You wanted Mukunda's position, but could not maintain it by merit. Return now to your earlier work as cook's assistant."

After this humbling incident, Master resumed toward Kumar a former attitude of unwonted indulgence. Who can solve the mystery of attraction? In Kumar our guru discovered a charming fount which did not spurt for the fellow disciples. Though the new boy was obviously Sri Yukteswar's favorite, I felt no dismay. Personal idiosyncrasies, possessed even by masters, lend a rich complexity to the pattern of life. My nature is seldom commandeered by a detail; I was seeking from Sri Yukteswar a more inaccessible benefit than an outward praise.

Kumar spoke venomously to me one day without reason; I was deeply hurt.

"Your head is swelling to the bursting point!" I added a warning whose truth I felt intuitively: "Unless you mend your ways, someday you will be asked to leave this ashram."

Laughing sarcastically, Kumar repeated my remark to our guru, who had just entered the room. Fully expecting to be scolded, I retired meekly to a corner.

"Maybe Mukunda is right." Master's reply to the boy came with unusual coldness. I escaped without castigation.

A year later, Kumar set out for a visit to his childhood home. He ignored the quiet disapproval of Sri Yukteswar, who never authoritatively controlled his disciples' movements. On the boy's return to Serampore in a few months, a change was unpleasantly apparent. Gone was the stately Kumar with serenely glowing face. Only an undistinguished peasant stood before us, one who had lately acquired a number of evil habits.

Master summoned me and brokenheartedly discussed the fact that the boy was now unsuited to the monastic hermitage life.

"Mukunda, I will leave it to you to instruct Kumar to leave the ashram tomorrow; I can't do it!" Tears stood in Sri Yukteswar's eyes, but he controlled himself quickly. "The boy would never have fallen to these depths had he listened to me and not gone away to mix with undesirable companions. He has rejected my protection; the callous world must be his guru still."

Kumar's departure brought me no elation; sadly I wondered how one with power to win a master's love could ever respond to cheaper allures. Enjoyment of wine and sex are rooted in the natural man, and require no delicacies of perception for their appreciation. Sense wiles are comparable to the evergreen oleander, fragrant with its multicolored flowers: every part of the plant is poisonous.

The land of healing lies within, radiant with that happiness blindly sought in a thousand misdirections.[19]

"Keen intelligence is two-edged," Master once remarked in reference to Kumar's brilliant mind. "It may be used constructively or destructively like a knife, either to cut the boil of ignorance, or to decapitate one's self. Intelligence is rightly guided only after the mind has acknowledged the inescapability of spiritual law."

My guru mixed freely with men and women disciples, treating all as his children. Perceiving their soul equality, he showed no distinction or partiality.

"In sleep, you do not know whether you are a man or a woman," he said. "Just as a man, impersonating a woman, does not become one, so the soul, impersonating both man and woman, has no sex. The soul is the pure, changeless image of God."

Sri Yukteswar never avoided or blamed women as objects of seduction. Men, he said, were also a temptation to women. I once inquired of my guru why a great ancient saint had called women "the door to hell."

"A girl must have proved very troublesome to his peace of mind in his early life," my guru answered causticly. "Otherwise he would have denounced, not woman, but some imperfection in his own self-control."

If a visitor dared to relate a suggestive story in the hermitage, Master would maintain an unresponsive silence. "Do not allow yourself to be thrashed by the provoking whip of a beautiful face," he told the disciples. "How can sense slaves enjoy the world? Its subtle flavors escape them while they grovel in primal mud. All nice discriminations are lost to the man of elemental lusts."

Students seeking to escape from the dualistic *maya* delusion received from Sri Yukteswar patient and understanding counsel.

"Just as the purpose of eating is to satisfy hunger, not greed, so the sex instinct is designed for the propagation of the species according to natural law, never for the kindling of insatiable longings," he said. "Destroy wrong desires now; otherwise they will follow you after the astral body is torn from its physical casing. Even when the flesh is weak, the mind should be constantly resistant. If temptation assails you with cruel force, overcome it by impersonal analysis and indomitable will. Every natural passion can be mastered.

"Conserve your powers. Be like the capacious ocean, absorbing within all the tributary rivers of the senses. Small yearnings are openings in the reservoir of your inner peace, permitting healing waters to be wasted in the desert soil of materialism. The forceful activating impulse of wrong desire is the greatest enemy to the happiness of man. Roam in the world as a lion of self-control; see that the frogs of weakness don't kick you around."

The devotee is finally freed from all instinctive compulsions. He transforms his need for human affection into aspiration for God alone, a love solitary because omnipresent.

Sri Yukteswar's mother lived in the Rana Mahal district of Benares where I had first visited my guru. Gracious and kindly, she was yet a woman of very decided opinions. I stood on her balcony one day and watched mother and son talking together. In his quiet, sensible way, Master was trying to convince her about something. He was apparently unsuccessful, for she shook her head with great vigor.

"Nay, nay, my son, go away now! Your wise words are not for me! I am not your disciple!"

Sri Yukteswar backed away without further argument, like a scolded child. I was touched at his great respect for his mother even in her unreasonable moods. She saw him only as her little boy, not as a sage. There was a charm about the trifling incident; it supplied a sidelight on my guru's unusual nature, inwardly humble and outwardly unbendable.

The monastic regulations do not allow a swami to retain connection with worldly ties after their formal severance. He cannot perform the ceremonial family rites which are obligatory on the householder. Yet Shankara, the ancient founder of the Swami Order, disregarded the injunctions. At the death of his beloved mother, he cremated her body with heavenly fire which he caused to spurt from his upraised hand.

Sri Yukteswar also ignored the restrictions, in a fashion less spectacular. When his mother passed on, he arranged the crematory services by the holy Ganges in Benares, and fed many Brahmins in conformance with age-old custom.

The *shastric* prohibitions were intended to help swamis overcome narrow identifications. Shankara and Sri Yukteswar had wholly merged their beings in the Impersonal Spirit; they needed no rescue by rule. Sometimes, too, a master purposely ignores a canon in order to uphold its principle as superior to and independent of form. Thus Jesus plucked ears of corn on the day of rest. To the inevitable critics he said: "The sabbath was made for man, and not man for the sabbath."[20]

Outside of the scriptures, seldom was a book honored by Sri Yukteswar's perusal. Yet he was invariably acquainted with the latest scientific discoveries and other advancements of knowledge. A brilliant conversationalist, he enjoyed an exchange of views on countless topics with his guests. My guru's ready wit and rollicking laugh enlivened every discussion. Often grave, Master was never gloomy. "To seek the Lord, one need not disfigure his face," he would remark. "Remember that finding God will mean the funeral of all sorrows."

Among the philosophers, professors, lawyers and scientists who came to the hermitage, a number arrived for their first visit with the expectation of meeting an orthodox religionist. A supercilious smile or a glance of amused tolerance occasionally betrayed that the newcomers anticipated nothing more than a few pious platitudes. Yet their reluctant departure would bring an expressed conviction that Sri Yukteswar had shown precise insight into their specialized fields.

My guru ordinarily was gentle and affable to guests; his welcome was given with charming cordiality. Yet inveterate egotists sometimes suffered an invigorating shock. They confronted in Master either a frigid indifference or a formidable opposition: ice or iron!

A noted chemist once crossed swords with Sri Yukteswar. The visitor would not admit the existence of God, inasmuch as science has devised no means of detecting Him.

"So you have inexplicably failed to isolate the Supreme Power in your test tubes!" Master's gaze was stern. "I recommend an unheard-of experiment. Examine your thoughts unremittingly for twenty-four hours. Then wonder no longer at God's absence."

A celebrated pundit received a similar jolt. With ostentatious zeal, the scholar shook the ashram rafters with scriptural lore. Resounding passages poured from the *Mahabharata,* the *Upanishads,*[21] the *bhasyas*[22] of Shankara.

"I am waiting to hear you." Sri Yukteswar's tone was inquiring, as though utter silence had reigned. The pundit was puzzled.

"Quotations there have been, in superabundance." Master's words convulsed me with mirth, as I squatted in my corner, at a respectful distance from the visitor. "But what original commentary can you supply, from the uniqueness of your particular life? What holy text have you absorbed and made your own? In what ways have these timeless truths renovated your nature? Are you content to be a hollow victrola, mechanically repeating the words of other men?"

"I give up!" The scholar's chagrin was comical. "I have no inner realization."

For the first time, perhaps, he understood that discerning placement of the comma does not atone for a spiritual coma.

"These bloodless pedants smell unduly of the lamp," my guru remarked after the departure of the chastened one. "They prefer philosophy to be a gentle intellectual setting-up exercise. Their elevated thoughts are carefully unrelated either to the crudity of outward action or to any scourging inner discipline!"

Master stressed on other occasions the futility of mere book learning.

"Do not confuse understanding with a larger vocabulary," he remarked. "Sacred writings are beneficial in stimulating desire for inward realization, if one stanza at a time is slowly assimilated. Continual intellectual study results in vanity and the false satisfaction of an undigested knowledge."

Sri Yukteswar related one of his own experiences in scriptural edification. The scene was a forest hermitage in eastern Bengal, where he observed the procedure of a renowned teacher, Dabru Ballav. His method, at once simple and difficult, was common in ancient India.

Dabru Ballav had gathered his disciples around him in the sylvan solitudes. The holy *Bhagavad Gita* was open before them. Steadfastly they looked at one passage for half an hour, then closed their eyes. Another half hour slipped away. The master gave a brief comment. Motionless, they meditated again for an hour. Finally the guru spoke.

"Have you understood?"

"Yes, sir." One in the group ventured this assertion.

"No; not fully. Seek the spiritual vitality that has given these words the power to rejuvenate India century after century." Another hour disappeared in silence. The master dismissed the students, and turned to Sri Yukteswar.

"Do you know the *Bhagavad Gita?*"

"No, sir, not really; though my eyes and mind have run through its pages many times."

"Thousands have replied to me differently!" The great sage smiled at Master in blessing. "If one busies himself with an outer display of scriptural wealth, what time is left for silent inward diving after the priceless pearls?"

Sri Yukteswar directed the study of his own disciples by the same intensive method of one-pointedness. "Wisdom is not assimilated with the eyes, but with the atoms," he said. "When your conviction of a truth is not merely in your brain but in your being, you may diffidently vouch for its meaning." He discouraged any tendency a student might have to construe book-knowledge as a necessary step to spiritual realization.

"The *rishis* wrote in one sentence profundities that commentating scholars busy themselves over for generations," he remarked. "Endless literary controversy is for sluggard minds. What more liberating thought than 'God is'-nay, 'God'?"

But man does not easily return to simplicity. It is seldom "God" for him, but rather learned pomposities. His ego is pleased, that he can grasp such erudition.

Men who were pridefully conscious of high worldly position were likely, in Master's presence, to add humility to their other possessions. A local magistrate once arrived for an interview at the seaside hermitage in Puri. The man, who held a reputation for ruthlessness, had it well within his power to oust us from the ashram. I cautioned my guru about the despotic possibilities. But he seated himself with an uncompromising air, and did not rise to greet the visitor. Slightly nervous, I squatted near the door. The man had to content himself with a wooden box; my guru did not request me to fetch a chair. There was no fulfillment of the magistrate's obvious expectation that his importance would be ceremoniously acknowledged.

A metaphysical discussion ensued. The guest blundered through misinterpretations of the scriptures. As his accuracy sank, his ire rose.

"Do you know that I stood first in the M. A. examination?" Reason had forsaken him, but he could still shout.

"Mr. Magistrate, you forget that this is not your courtroom," Master replied evenly. "From your childish remarks I would have surmised that your college career was unremarkable. A university degree, in any case, is not remotely related to Vedic realization. Saints are not produced in batches every semester like accountants."

After a stunned silence, the visitor laughed heartily.

"This is my first encounter with a heavenly magistrate," he said. Later he made a formal request, couched in the legal terms which were evidently part and parcel of his being, to be accepted as a "probationary" disciple.

My guru personally attended to the details connected with the management of his property. Unscrupulous persons on various occasions attempted to secure possession of Master's ancestral land. With determination and even by instigating lawsuits, Sri Yukteswar outwitted every opponent. He underwent these painful experiences from a desire never to be a begging guru, or a burden on his disciples.

His financial independence was one reason why my alarmingly outspoken Master was innocent of the cunnings of diplomacy. Unlike those teachers who have to flatter their supporters, my guru was impervious to the influences, open or subtle, of others' wealth. Never did I hear him ask or even hint for money for any purpose. His hermitage training was given free and freely to all disciples.

An insolent court deputy arrived one day at the Serampore ashram to serve Sri Yukteswar with a legal summons. A disciple named

Kanai and myself were also present. The officer's attitude toward Master was offensive.

"It will do you good to leave the shadows of your hermitage and breathe the honest air of a courtroom." The deputy grinned contemptuously. I could not contain myself.

"Another word of your impudence and you will be on the floor!" I advanced threateningly.

"You wretch!" Kanai's shout was simultaneous with my own. "Dare you bring your blasphemies into this sacred ashram?"

But Master stood protectingly in front of his abuser. "Don't get excited over nothing. This man is only doing his rightful duty."

The officer, dazed at his varying reception, respectfully offered a word of apology and sped away.

Amazing it was to find that a master with such a fiery will could be so calm within. He fitted the Vedic definition of a man of God: "Softer than the flower, where kindness is concerned; stronger than the thunder, where principles are at stake."

There are always those in this world who, in Browning's words, "endure no light, being themselves obscure." An outsider occasionally berated Sri Yukteswar for an imaginary grievance. My imperturbable guru listened politely, analyzing himself to see if any shred of truth lay within the denunciation. These scenes would bring to my mind one of Master's inimitable observations: "Some people try to be tall by cutting off the heads of others!"

The unfailing composure of a saint is impressive beyond any sermon. "He that is slow to anger is better than the mighty; and he that ruleth his spirit than he that taketh a city."[23]

I often reflected that my majestic Master could easily have been an emperor or world-shaking warrior had his mind been centered on fame or worldly achievement. He had chosen instead to storm

167

those inner citadels of wrath and egotism whose fall is the height of a man.

[1] "Worship of Durga." This is the chief festival of the Bengali year and lasts for nine days around the end of September. Immediately following is the ten-day festival of Dashahara ("the One who removes ten sins"-three of body, three of mind, four of speech). Both pujas are sacred to Durga, literally "the Inaccessible," an aspect of Divine Mother, Shakti, the female creative force personified.

[2] Sri Yukteswar was born on May 10, 1855.

[3] Yukteswar means "united to God." Giri is a classificatory distinction of one of the ten ancient Swami branches. Sri means "holy"; it is not a name but a title of respect.

[4] Literally, "to direct together." Samadhi is a superconscious state of ecstasy in which the yogi perceives the identity of soul and Spirit.

[5] Snoring, according to physiologists, is an indication of utter relaxation (to the oblivious practitioner, solely).

[6] Dhal is a thick soup made from split peas or other pulses. Channa is a cheese of fresh curdled milk, cut into squares and curried with potatoes.

[7] The omnipresent powers of a yogi, whereby he sees, hears, tastes, smells, and feels his oneness in creation without the use of sensory organs, have been described as follows in the Taittiriya Aranyaka: "The blind man pierced the pearl; the fingerless put a thread into it; the neckless wore it; and the tongueless praised it."

[8] The cobra swiftly strikes at any moving object within its range. Complete immobility is usually one's sole hope of safety.

[9] Lahiri Mahasaya actually said "Priya" (first or given name), not "Yukteswar" (monastic name, not received by my guru during Lahiri Mahasaya's lifetime). (See page 109.) Yukteswar" is substituted here, and in a few other places in this book, in order to avoid the confusion, to reader, of two names.

[10] "Therefore I say unto you, What things soever ye desire, when ye pray, believe that ye receive them, and ye shall have them."-Mark 11:24. Masters who possess the Divine Vision are fully able to transfer their realizations to

advanced disciples, as Lahiri Mahasaya did for Sri Yukteswar on this occasion.

[11]"And one of them smote the servant of the high priest, and cut off his right ear. And Jesus answered and said, Suffer ye thus far. And he touched his ear and healed him."-Luke 22:50-51.

[12]"Give not that which is holy unto the dogs, neither cast ye your pearls before swine, lest they trample them under their feet, and turn again and rend you."-Matthew 7:6.

[13] Disciples; from Sanskrit verb root, "to serve."

[14] He was once ill in Kashmir, when I was absent from him. (See page 209.)

[15] A courageous medical man, Charles Robert Richet, awarded the Nobel Prize in physiology, wrote as follows: "Metaphysics is not yet officially a science, recognized as such. But it is going to be. . . . At Edinburgh, I was able to affirm before 100 physiologists that our five senses are not our only means of knowledge and that a fragment of reality sometimes reaches the intelligence in other ways. . . . Because a fact is rare is no reason that it does not exist. Because a study is difficult, is that a reason for not understanding it? . . . Those who have railed at metaphysics as an occult science will be as ashamed of themselves as those who railed at chemistry on the ground that pursuit of the philosopher's stone was illusory. . . . In the matter of principles there are only those of Lavoisier, Claude Bernard, and Pasteur-the experimental everywhere and always. Greetings, then, to the new science which is going to change the orientation of human thought."

[16] Samadhi: perfect union of the individualized soul with the Infinite Spirit.

[17] The subconsciously guided rationalizations of the mind are utterly different from the infallible guidance of truth which issues from the superconsciousness. Led by French scientists of the Sorbonne, Western thinkers are beginning to investigate the possibility of divine perception in man.

"For the past twenty years, students of psychology, influenced by Freud, gave all their time to searching the subconscious realms," Rabbi Israel H. Levinthal pointed out in 1929. "It is true that the subconscious reveals much of the mystery that can explain human actions, but not all of our actions. It can explain the abnormal, but not deeds that are above the normal. The latest psychology, sponsored by the French schools, has discovered a new region in man, which it terms the superconscious. In contrast to the subconscious which represents the submerged currents of our nature, it reveals the heights to which our nature can reach. Man represents a triple, not a double, personality; our conscious and subconscious being is crowned by a superconsciousness. Many years ago the English psychologist, F. W. H. Myers, suggested that 'hidden in the deep of our being is a rubbish heap as well as a treasure house.' In contrast to the psychology that centers all its researches on the subconscious in man's nature, this new psychology of the superconscious focuses its attention upon the treasure-house, the region that alone can explain the great, unselfish, heroic deeds of men."

[18] Jnana, wisdom, and bhakti, devotion: two of the main paths to God.

[19] "Man in his waking state puts forth innumerable efforts for experiencing sensual pleasures; when the entire group of sensory organs is fatigued, he forgets even the pleasure on hand and goes to sleep in order to enjoy rest in the soul, his own nature," Shankara, the great Vedantist, has written. "Ultra-sensual bliss is thus extremely easy of attainment and is far superior to sense delights which always end in disgust."

[20] Mark 2:27.

[21] The Upanishads or Vedanta (literally, "end of the Vedas"), occur in certain parts of the Vedas as essential summaries. The Upanishads furnish the doctrinal basis of the Hindu religion. They received the following tribute from Schopenhauer: "How entirely does the Upanishad breathe throughout the holy spirit of the Vedas! How is everyone who has become familiar with that incomparable book stirred by that spirit to the very depths of his soul! From every sentence deep, original, and sublime thoughts arise, and the whole is pervaded by a high and holy and earnest spirit. . . . The access to the Vedas by means of the Upanishads is in my eyes the greatest privilege this century may claim before all previous centuries."

[22] Commentaries. Shankara peerlessly expounded the Upanishads.

[23] Proverbs 16:32.

## CHAPTER 14

# *An Experience in Cosmic Consciousness*

"I am here, Guruji." My shamefacedness spoke more eloquently for me.

"Let us go to the kitchen and find something to eat." Sri Yukteswar's manner was as natural as if hours and not days had separated us.

"Master, I must have disappointed you by my abrupt departure from my duties here; I thought you might be angry with me."

"No, of course not! Wrath springs only from thwarted desires. I do not expect anything from others, so their actions cannot be in opposition to wishes of mine. I would not use you for my own ends; I am happy only in your own true happiness."

"Sir, one hears of divine love in a vague way, but for the first time I am having a concrete example in your angelic self! In the world, even a father does not easily forgive his son if he leaves his parent's business without warning. But you show not the slightest vexation, though you must have been put to great inconvenience by the many unfinished tasks I left behind."

We looked into each other's eyes, where tears were shining. A blissful wave engulfed me; I was conscious that the Lord, in the form of my guru, was expanding the small ardors of my heart into the incompressible reaches of cosmic love.

A few mornings later I made my way to Master's empty sitting room. I planned to meditate, but my laudable purpose was unshared by disobedient thoughts. They scattered like birds before the hunter.

"Mukunda!" Sri Yukteswar's voice sounded from a distant inner balcony.

I felt as rebellious as my thoughts. "Master always urges me to meditate," I muttered to myself. "He should not disturb me when he knows why I came to his room."

He summoned me again; I remained obstinately silent. The third time his tone held rebuke.

"Sir, I am meditating," I shouted protestingly.

"I know how you are meditating," my guru called out, "with your mind distributed like leaves in a storm! Come here to me."

Snubbed and exposed, I made my way sadly to his side.

"Poor boy, the mountains couldn't give what you wanted." Master spoke caressively, comfortingly. His calm gaze was unfathomable. "Your heart's desire shall be fulfilled."

Sri Yukteswar seldom indulged in riddles; I was bewildered. He struck gently on my chest above the heart.

My body became immovably rooted; breath was drawn out of my lungs as if by some huge magnet. Soul and mind instantly lost their physical bondage, and streamed out like a fluid piercing light from my every pore. The flesh was as though dead, yet in my intense awareness I knew that never before had I been fully alive. My sense of identity was no longer narrowly confined to a body, but embraced the circumambient atoms. People on distant streets seemed to be moving gently over my own remote periphery. The roots of plants and trees appeared through a dim transparency of the soil; I discerned the inward flow of their sap.

The whole vicinity lay bare before me. My ordinary frontal vision was now changed to a vast spherical sight, simultaneously all-perceptive. Through the back of my head I saw men strolling far down Rai Ghat Road, and noticed also a white cow who was leisurely approaching. When she reached the space in front of the open ashram gate, I observed her with my two physical eyes. As she passed by, behind the brick wall, I saw her clearly still.

All objects within my panoramic gaze trembled and vibrated like quick motion pictures. My body, Master's, the pillared courtyard, the furniture and floor, the trees and sunshine, occasionally became violently agitated, until all melted into a luminescent sea; even as sugar crystals, thrown into a glass of water, dissolve after being shaken. The unifying light alternated with materializations of form, the metamorphoses revealing the law of cause and effect in creation.

An oceanic joy broke upon calm endless shores of my soul. The Spirit of God, I realized, is exhaustless Bliss; His body is countless tissues of light. A swelling glory within me began to envelop towns, continents, the earth, solar and stellar systems, tenuous nebulae, and floating universes. The entire cosmos, gently luminous, like a city seen afar at night, glimmered within the infinitude of my being. The sharply etched global outlines faded somewhat at the farthest edges; there I could see a mellow radiance, ever-undiminished. It was indescribably subtle; the planetary pictures were formed of a grosser light.

The divine dispersion of rays poured from an Eternal Source, blazing into galaxies, transfigured with ineffable auras. Again and again I saw the creative beams condense into constellations, then resolve into sheets of transparent flame. By rhythmic reversion, sextillion worlds passed into diaphanous luster; fire became firmament.

I cognized the center of the empyrean as a point of intuitive perception in my heart. Irradiating splendor issued from my nucleus to every part of the universal structure. Blissful *amrita,* the nectar of immortality, pulsed through me with a quicksilver-like fluidity. The creative voice of God I heard resounding as *Aum,*[1] the vibration of the Cosmic Motor.

Suddenly the breath returned to my lungs. With a disappointment almost unbearable, I realized that my infinite immensity was lost. Once more I was limited to the humiliating cage of a body, not easily accommodative to the Spirit. Like a prodigal child, I had run away from my macrocosmic home and imprisoned myself in a narrow microcosm.

My guru was standing motionless before me; I started to drop at his holy feet in gratitude for the experience in cosmic consciousness which I had long passionately sought. He held me upright, and spoke calmly, unpretentiously.

"You must not get overdrunk with ecstasy. Much work yet remains for you in the world. Come; let us sweep the balcony floor; then we shall walk by the Ganges."

I fetched a broom; Master, I knew, was teaching me the secret of balanced living. The soul must stretch over the cosmogonic abysses, while the body performs its daily duties. When we set out later for a stroll, I was still entranced in unspeakable rapture. I saw our bodies as two astral pictures, moving over a road by the river whose essence was sheer light.

"It is the Spirit of God that actively sustains every form and force in the universe; yet He is transcendental and aloof in the blissful uncreated void beyond the worlds of vibratory phenomena," [2] Master explained. "Saints who realize their divinity even while in the flesh know a similar twofold existence. Conscientiously engaging in earthly work, they yet remain immersed in an inward beatitude. The Lord has created all men from the limitless joy of His being. Though they are painfully cramped by the body, God nevertheless expects that souls made in His image shall ultimately rise above all sense identifications and reunite with Him."

The cosmic vision left many permanent lessons. By daily stilling my thoughts, I could win release from the delusive conviction that my body was a mass of flesh and bones, traversing the hard soil of matter. The breath and the restless mind, I saw, were like storms which lashed the ocean of light into waves of material forms-earth, sky, human beings, animals, birds, trees. No perception of the Infinite as One Light could be had except by calming those storms. As often as I silenced the two natural tumults, I beheld the multitudinous waves of creation melt into one lucent sea, even as the waves of the ocean, their tempests subsiding, serenely dissolve into unity.

A master bestows the divine experience of cosmic consciousness when his disciple, by meditation, has strengthened his mind to a degree where the vast vistas would not overwhelm him. The experience can never be given through one's mere intellectual willingness or open-mindedness. Only adequate enlargement by yoga practice and devotional *bhakti* can prepare the mind to absorb the liberating shock of omnipresence. It comes with a natural inevitability to the sincere devotee. His intense craving begins to pull at God with an irresistible force. The Lord, as the Cosmic Vision, is drawn by the seeker's magnetic ardor into his range of consciousness.

I wrote, in my later years, the following poem, "Samadhi," endeavoring to convey the glory of its cosmic state:


*Vanished the veils of light and shade,*

*Lifted every vapor of sorrow,*

*Sailed away all dawns of fleeting joy,*

*Gone the dim sensory mirage.*

*Love, hate, health, disease, life, death,*

*Perished these false shadows on the screen of duality.*

*Waves of laughter, scyllas of sarcasm, melancholic whirlpools,*

*Melting in the vast sea of bliss.*

*The storm of maya stilled*

*By magic wand of intuition deep.*

*The universe, forgotten dream, subconsciously lurks,*

*Ready to invade my newly-wakened memory divine.*

## Master of Kriya Yoga

*I live without the cosmic shadow,*

*But it is not, bereft of me;*

*As the sea exists without the waves,*

*But they breathe not without the sea.*

*Dreams, wakings, states of deep turia sleep,*

*Present, past, future, no more for me,*

*But ever-present, all-flowing I, I, everywhere.*

*Planets, stars, stardust, earth,*

*Volcanic bursts of doomsday cataclysms,*

*Creation's molding furnace,*

*Glaciers of silent x-rays, burning electron floods,*

*Thoughts of all men, past, present, to come,*

*Every blade of grass, myself, mankind,*

*Each particle of universal dust,*

*Anger, greed, good, bad, salvation, lust,*

*I swallowed, transmuted all*

*Into a vast ocean of blood of my own one Being!*

*Smoldering joy, oft-puffed by meditation*

*Blinding my tearful eyes,*

*Burst into immortal flames of bliss,*

*Consumed my tears, my frame, my all.*

*Thou art I, I am Thou,*

*Knowing, Knower, Known, as One!*

## The Essence of Kriya Yoga

*Tranquilled, unbroken thrill, eternally living, ever-new peace!*

*Enjoyable beyond imagination of expectancy, samadhi bliss!*

*Not an unconscious state*

*Or mental chloroform without wilful return,*

*Samadhi but extends my conscious realm*

*Beyond limits of the mortal frame*

*To farthest boundary of eternity*

*Where I, the Cosmic Sea,*

*Watch the little ego floating in Me.*

*The sparrow, each grain of sand, fall not without My sight.*

*All space floats like an iceberg in My mental sea.*

*Colossal Container, I, of all things made.*

*By deeper, longer, thirsty, guru-given meditation*

*Comes this celestial samadhi.*

*Mobile murmurs of atoms are heard,*

*The dark earth, mountains, vales, lo! molten liquid!*

*Flowing seas change into vapors of nebulae!*

*Aum blows upon vapors, opening wondrously their veils,*

*Oceans stand revealed, shining electrons,*

*Till, at last sound of the cosmic drum,*

*Vanish the grosser lights into eternal rays*

*Of all-pervading bliss.*

*From joy I came, for joy I live, in sacred joy I melt.*

*Ocean of mind, I drink all creation's waves.*

*Four veils of solid, liquid, vapor, light,*

*Lift aright.*

*Myself, in everything, enters the Great Myself.*

*Gone forever, fitful, flickering shadows of mortal memory.*

*Spotless is my mental sky, below, ahead, and high above.*

*Eternity and I, one united ray.*

*A tiny bubble of laughter, I*

*Am become the Sea of Mirth Itself.*

Sri Yukteswar taught me how to summon the blessed experience at will, and also how to transmit it to others if their intuitive channels were developed. For months I entered the ecstatic union, comprehending why the *Upanishads* say God is *rasa,* "the most relishable." One day, however, I took a problem to Master.

"I want to know, sir - when shall I find God?"

"You have found Him."

"O no, sir, I don't think so!"

My guru was smiling. "I am sure you aren't expecting a venerable Personage, adorning a throne in some antiseptic corner of the cosmos! I see, however, that you are imagining that the possession of miraculous powers is knowledge of God. One might have the whole universe, and find the Lord elusive still! Spiritual advancement is not measured by one's outward powers, but only by the depth of his bliss in meditation.

"*Ever-new Joy is God.* He is inexhaustible; as you continue your meditations during the years, He will beguile you with an infinite ingenuity. Devotees like yourself who have found the way to God never dream of exchanging Him for any other happiness; He is seductive beyond thought of competition.

"How quickly we weary of earthly pleasures! Desire for material things is endless; man is never satisfied completely, and pursues one goal after another. The 'something else' he seeks is the Lord, who alone can grant lasting joy.

"Outward longings drive us from the Eden within; they offer false pleasures which only impersonate soul-happiness. The lost paradise is quickly regained through divine meditation. As God is unanticipatory Ever-Newness, we never tire of Him. Can we be surfeited with bliss, delightfully varied throughout eternity?"

"I understand now, sir, why saints call the Lord unfathomable. Even everlasting life could not suffice to appraise Him."

"That is true; but He is also near and dear. After the mind has been cleared by *Kriya Yoga* of sensory obstacles, meditation furnishes a twofold proof of God. Ever-new joy is evidence of His existence, convincing to our very atoms. Also, in meditation one finds His instant guidance, His adequate response to every difficulty."

"I see, Guruji; you have solved my problem." I smiled gratefully. "I do realize now that I have found God, for whenever the joy of meditation has returned subconsciously during my active hours, I have been subtly directed to adopt the right course in everything, even details."

"Human life is beset with sorrow until we know how to tune in with the Divine Will, whose 'right course' is often baffling to the egoistic intelligence. God bears the burden of the cosmos; He alone can give unerring counsel."

---

[1] "In the beginning was the Word, and the Word was with God, and the Word was God."-John 1:1

[2] "For the Father judgeth no man, but hath committed all judgment unto the Son."-John 5:22. "No man hath seen God at any time; the only begotten Son, which is in the bosom of the Father, he hath declared him."-John 1:18. "Verily, verily, I say unto you, he that believeth on me, the works that I do shall he do also; and greater works than these shall he do; because I go unto my Father."-John 14:12. "But the Comforter, which is the Holy Ghost, whom the Father will send in my name, he shall teach you all things, and bring all things to your remembrance, whatsoever I have said to you."-John 14:26.

These Biblical words refer to the threefold nature of God as Father, Son, Holy Ghost (Sat, Tat, Aum in the Hindu scriptures). God the Father is the Absolute, Unmanifested, existing beyond vibratory creation. God the Son is the Christ Consciousness (Brahma or Kutastha Chaitanya) existing within vibratory creation; this Christ Consciousness is the "only begotten" or sole reflection of the Uncreated Infinite. Its outward manifestation or "witness" is Aum or Holy Ghost, the divine, creative, invisible power which structures all creation through vibration. Aum the blissful Comforter is heard in meditation and reveals to the devotee the ultimate Truth.

## CHAPTER 19

# *My Master, in Calcutta, Appears in Serampore*

"I am often beset by atheistic doubts. Yet a torturing surmise sometimes haunts me: may not untapped soul possibilities exist? Is man not missing his real destiny if he fails to explore them?"

These remarks of Dijen Babu, my roommate at the *Panthi* boardinghouse, were called forth by my invitation that he meet my guru.

"Sri Yukteswarji will initiate you into *Kriya Yoga*," I replied. "It calms the dualistic turmoil by a divine inner certainty."

That evening Dijen accompanied me to the hermitage. In Master's presence my friend received such spiritual peace that he was soon a constant visitor. The trivial preoccupations of daily life are not enough for man; wisdom too is a native hunger. In Sri Yukteswar's words Dijen found an incentive to those attempts-first painful, then effortlessly liberating-to locate a realer self within his bosom than the humiliating ego of a temporary birth, seldom ample enough for the Spirit.

As Dijen and I were both pursuing the A.B. course at Serampore College, we got into the habit of walking together to the ashram as soon as classes were over. We would often see Sri Yukteswar standing on his second-floor balcony, welcoming our approach with a smile.

One afternoon Kanai, a young hermitage resident, met Dijen and me at the door with disappointing news.

"Master is not here; he was summoned to Calcutta by an urgent note."

The following day I received a post card from my guru. "I shall leave Calcutta Wednesday morning," he had written. "You and Dijen meet the nine o'clock train at Serampore station."

About eight-thirty on Wednesday morning, a telepathic message from Sri Yukteswar flashed insistently to my mind: "I am delayed; don't meet the nine o'clock train."

I conveyed the latest instructions to Dijen, who was already dressed for departure.

"You and your intuition!" My friend's voice was edged in scorn. "I prefer to trust Master's written word."

I shrugged my shoulders and seated myself with quiet finality. Muttering angrily, Dijen made for the door and closed it noisily behind him.

As the room was rather dark, I moved nearer to the window overlooking the street. The scant sunlight suddenly increased to an intense brilliancy in which the iron-barred window completely vanished. Against this dazzling background appeared the clearly materialized figure of Sri Yukteswar!

Bewildered to the point of shock, I rose from my chair and knelt before him. With my customary gesture of respectful greeting at my guru's feet, I touched his shoes. These were a pair familiar to me, of orange-dyed canvas, soled with rope. His ocher swami cloth brushed against me; I distinctly felt not only the texture of his robe, but also the gritty surface of the shoes, and the pressure of his toes within them. Too much astounded to utter a word, I stood up and gazed at him questioningly.

"I was pleased that you got my telepathic message." Master's voice was calm, entirely normal. "I have now finished my business in Calcutta, and shall arrive in Serampore by the ten o'clock train."

As I still stared mutely, Sri Yukteswar went on, "This is not an apparition, but my flesh and blood form. I have been divinely commanded to give you this experience, rare to achieve on earth. Meet me at the station; you and Dijen will see me coming toward you, dressed as I am now. I shall be preceded by a fellow passenger-a little boy carrying a silver jug."

My guru placed both hands on my head, with a murmured blessing. As he concluded with the words, *"Taba asi,"*[1] I heard a peculiar rumbling sound.[2] His body began to melt gradually within the piercing light. First his feet and legs vanished, then his torso and head, like a scroll being rolled up. To the very last, I could feel his fingers resting lightly on my hair. The effulgence faded; nothing remained before me but the barred window and a pale stream of sunlight.

I remained in a half-stupor of confusion, questioning whether I had not been the victim of a hallucination. A crestfallen Dijen soon entered the room.

"Master was not on the nine o'clock train, nor even the nine-thirty." My friend made his announcement with a slightly apologetic air.

"Come then; I know he will arrive at ten o'clock." I took Dijen's hand and rushed him forcibly along with me, heedless of his protests. In about ten minutes we entered the station, where the train was already puffing to a halt.

"The whole train is filled with the light of Master's aura! He is there!" I exclaimed joyfully.

"You dream so?" Dijen laughed mockingly.

"Let us wait here." I told my friend details of the way in which our guru would approach us. As I finished my description, Sri Yukteswar came into view, wearing the same clothes I had seen a short time earlier. He walked slowly in the wake of a small lad bearing a silver jug.

For a moment a wave of cold fear passed through me, at the unprecedented strangeness of my experience. I felt the materialistic, twentieth-century world slipping from me; was I back in the ancient days when Jesus appeared before Peter on the sea?

As Sri Yukteswar, a modern Yogi-Christ, reached the spot where Dijen and I were speechlessly rooted, Master smiled at my friend and remarked:

"I sent you a message too, but you were unable to grasp it."

Dijen was silent, but glared at me suspiciously. After we had escorted our guru to his hermitage, my friend and I proceeded toward Serampore College. Dijen halted in the street, indignation streaming from his every pore.

"So! Master sent me a message! Yet you concealed it! I demand an explanation!"

"Can I help it if your mental mirror oscillates with such restlessness that you cannot register our guru's instructions?" I retorted.

The anger vanished from Dijen's face. "I see what you mean," he said ruefully. "But please explain how you could know about the child with the jug."

By the time I had finished the story of Master's phenomenal appearance at the boardinghouse that morning, my friend and I had reached Serampore College.

"The account I have just heard of our guru's powers," Dijen said, "makes me feel that any university in the world is only a kindergarten."

---

[1] The Bengali "Good-by"; literally, it is a hopeful paradox: "Then I come."

[2] The characteristic sound of dematerialization of bodily atoms.

**CHAPTER 23**

# I Receive My University Degree

"You ignore your textbook assignments in philosophy. No doubt you are depending on an unlaborious 'intuition' to get you through the examinations. But unless you apply yourself in a more scholarly manner, I shall see to it that you don't pass this course."

Professor D. C. Ghoshal of Serampore College was addressing me sternly. If I failed to pass his final written classroom test, I would be ineligible to take the conclusive examinations. These are formulated by the faculty of Calcutta University, which numbers Serampore College among its affiliated branches. A student in Indian universities who is unsuccessful in one subject in the A.B. finals must be examined anew in *all* his subjects the following year.

My instructors at Serampore College usually treated me with kindness, not untinged by an amused tolerance. "Mukunda is a bit over-drunk with religion." Thus summing me up, they tactfully spared me the embarrassment of answering classroom questions; they trusted the final written tests to eliminate me from the list of A.B. candidates. The judgment passed by my fellow students was expressed in their nickname for me-"Mad Monk."

I took an ingenious step to nullify Professor Ghoshal's threat to me of failure in philosophy. When the results of the final tests were about to be publicly announced, I asked a classmate to accompany me to the professor's study.

"Come along; I want a witness," I told my companion. "I shall be very much disappointed if I have not succeeded in outwitting the instructor."

Professor Ghoshal shook his head after I had inquired what rating he had given my paper.

"You are not among those who have passed," he said in triumph. He hunted through a large pile on his desk. "Your paper isn't here at all; you have failed, in any case, through non-appearance at the examination."

I chuckled. "Sir, I was there. May I look through the stack myself?"

The professor, nonplused, gave his permission; I quickly found my paper, where I had carefully omitted any identification mark except my roll call number. Unwarned by the "red flag" of my name, the instructor had given a high rating to my answers even though they were unembellished by textbook quotations.[1]

Seeing through my trick, he now thundered, "Sheer brazen luck!" He added hopefully, "You are sure to fail in the A.B. finals."

For the tests in my other subjects, I received some coaching, particularly from my dear friend and cousin, Prabhas Chandra Ghose,[2] son of my Uncle Sarada. I staggered painfully but successfully-with the lowest possible passing marks-through all my final tests.

Now, after four years of college, I was eligible to sit for the A.B. examinations. Nevertheless, I hardly expected to avail myself of the privilege. The Serampore College finals were child's play compared to the stiff ones which would be set by Calcutta University for the A.B. degree. My almost daily visits to Sri Yukteswar had left me little time to enter the college halls. There it was my presence rather than my absence that brought forth ejaculations of amazement from my classmates!

My customary routine was to set out on my bicycle about nine-thirty in the morning. In one hand I would carry an offering for my guru-a few flowers from the garden of my *Panthi* boardinghouse. Greeting me affably, Master would invite me to lunch. I invariably accepted with alacrity, glad to banish the thought of college for the day. After hours with Sri Yukteswar, listening to his incomparable flow of wisdom, or helping with ashram duties, I would reluctantly depart around midnight for the *Panthi*.

Occasionally I stayed all night with my guru, so happily engrossed in his conversation that I scarcely noticed when darkness changed into dawn.

One night about eleven o'clock, as I was putting on my shoes[3] in preparation for the ride to the boardinghouse, Master questioned me gravely.

"When do your A.B. examinations start?"

"Five days hence, sir."

"I hope you are in readiness for them."

Transfixed with alarm, I held one shoe in the air. "Sir," I protested, "you know how my days have been passed with you rather than with the professors. How can I enact a farce by appearing for those difficult finals?"

Sri Yukteswar's eyes were turned piercingly on mine. "You must appear." His tone was coldly peremptory. "We should not give cause for your father and other relatives to criticize your preference for ashram life. Just promise me that you will be present for the examinations; answer them the best way you can."

Uncontrollable tears were coursing down my face. I felt that Master's command was unreasonable, and that his interest was, to say the least, belated.

"I will appear if you wish it," I said amidst sobs. "But no time remains for proper preparation." Under my breath I muttered, "I will fill up the sheets with your teachings in answer to the questions!"

When I entered the hermitage the following day at my usual hour, I presented my bouquet with a certain mournful solemnity. Sri Yukteswar laughed at my woebegone air.

"Mukunda, has the Lord ever failed you, at an examination or elsewhere?"

"No, sir," I responded warmly. Grateful memories came in a revivifying flood.

"Not laziness but burning zeal for God has prevented you from seeking college honors," my guru said kindly. After a silence, he quoted, "'Seek ye first the kingdom of God, and His righteousness; and all these things shall be added unto you.'"[4]

For the thousandth time, I felt my burdens lifted in Master's presence. When we had finished our early lunch, he suggested that I return to the *Panthi.*

"Does your friend, Romesh Chandra Dutt, still live in your boardinghouse?"

"Yes, sir."

"Get in touch with him; the Lord will inspire him to help you with the examinations."

"Very well, sir; but Romesh is unusually busy. He is the honor man in our class, and carries a heavier course than the others."

Master waved aside my objections. "Romesh will find time for you. Now go."

I bicycled back to the *Panthi.* The first person I met in the boardinghouse compound was the scholarly Romesh. As though his days were quite free, he obligingly agreed to my diffident request.

"Of course; I am at your service." He spent several hours of that afternoon and of succeeding days in coaching me in my various subjects.

"I believe many questions in English literature will be centered in the route of Childe Harold," he told me. "We must get an atlas at once."

I hastened to the home of my Uncle Sarada and borrowed an atlas. Romesh marked the European map at the places visited by Byron's romantic traveler.

A few classmates had gathered around to listen to the tutoring. "Romesh is advising you wrongly," one of them commented to me at the end of a session. "Usually only fifty per cent of the questions are about the books; the other half will involve the authors' lives."

When I sat for the examination in English literature the following day, my first glance at the questions caused tears of gratitude to pour forth, wetting my paper. The classroom monitor came to my desk and made a sympathetic inquiry.

"My guru foretold that Romesh would help me," I explained. "Look; the very questions dictated to me by Romesh are here on the examination sheet! Fortunately for me, there are very few questions this year on English authors, whose lives are wrapped in deep mystery so far as I am concerned!"

My boardinghouse was in an uproar when I returned. The boys who had been ridiculing Romesh's method of coaching looked at me in awe, almost deafening me with congratulations. During the week of the examinations, I spent many hours with Romesh, who formulated questions that he thought were likely to be set by the professors. Day by day, Romesh's questions appeared in almost the same form on the examination sheets.

The news was widely circulated in the college that something resembling a miracle was occurring, and that success seemed probable for the absent-minded "Mad Monk." I made no attempt to hide the facts of the case. The local professors were powerless to alter the questions, which had been arranged by Calcutta University.

Thinking over the examination in English literature, I realized one morning that I had made a serious error. One section of the questions had been divided into two parts of A or B, and C or D.

Instead of answering one question from each part, I had carelessly answered both questions in Group I, and had failed to consider anything in Group II. The best mark I could score in that paper would be 33, three less than the passing mark of 36. I rushed to Master and poured out my troubles.

"Sir, I have made an unpardonable blunder. I don't deserve the divine blessings through Romesh; I am quite unworthy."

"Cheer up, Mukunda." Sri Yukteswar's tones were light and unconcerned. He pointed to the blue vault of the heavens. "It is more possible for the sun and moon to interchange their positions in space than it is for you to fail in getting your degree!"

I left the hermitage in a more tranquil mood, though it seemed mathematically inconceivable that I could pass. I looked once or twice apprehensively into the sky; the Lord of Day appeared to be securely anchored in his customary orbit!

As I reached the *Panthi,* I overheard a classmate's remark: "I have just learned that this year, for the first time, the required passing mark in English literature has been lowered."

I entered the boy's room with such speed that he looked up in alarm. I questioned him eagerly.

"Long-haired monk," he said laughingly, "why this sudden interest in scholastic matters? Why cry in the eleventh hour? But it is true that the passing mark has just been lowered to 33 points."

A few joyous leaps took me into my own room, where I sank to my knees and praised the mathematical perfections of my Divine Father.

Every day I thrilled with the consciousness of a spiritual presence that I clearly felt to be guiding me through Romesh. A significant incident occurred in connection with the examination in Bengali. Romesh, who had touched little on that subject, called me back one morning as I was leaving the boardinghouse on my way to the examination hall.

"There is Romesh shouting for you," a classmate said to me impatiently. "Don't return; we shall be late at the hall."

Ignoring the advice, I ran back to the house.

"The Bengali examination is usually easily passed by our Bengali boys," Romesh told me. "But I have just had a hunch that this year the professors have planned to massacre the students by asking questions from our ancient literature." My friend then briefly outlined two stories from the life of Vidyasagar, a renowned philanthropist.

I thanked Romesh and quickly bicycled to the college hall. The examination sheet in Bengali proved to contain two parts. The first instruction was: "Write two instances of the charities of Vidyasagar." As I transferred to the paper the lore that I had so recently acquired, I whispered a few words of thanksgiving that I had heeded Romesh's last-minute summons. Had I been ignorant of Vidyasagar's benefactions to mankind (including ultimately myself), I could not have passed the Bengali examination. Failing in one subject, I would have been forced to stand examination anew in all subjects the following year. Such a prospect was understandably abhorrent.

The second instruction on the sheet read: "Write an essay in Bengali on the life of the man who has most inspired you." Gentle reader, I need not inform you what man I chose for my theme. As I covered page after page with praise of my guru, I smiled to realize that my muttered prediction was coming true: "I will fill up the sheets with your teachings!"

I had not felt inclined to question Romesh about my course in philosophy. Trusting my long training under Sri Yukteswar, I safely disregarded the textbook explanations. The highest mark given to any of my papers was the one in philosophy. My score in all other subjects was just barely within the passing mark.

It is a pleasure to record that my unselfish friend Romesh received his own degree *cum laude.*

Father was wreathed in smiles at my graduation. "I hardly thought you would pass, Mukunda," he confessed. "You spend so much time with your guru." Master had indeed correctly detected the unspoken criticism of my father.

For years I had been uncertain that I would ever see the day when an A.B. would follow my name. I seldom use the title without reflecting that it was a divine gift, conferred on me for reasons somewhat obscure. Occasionally I hear college men remark that very little of their crammed knowledge remained with them after graduation. That admission consoles me a bit for my undoubted academic deficiencies.

On the day I received my degree from Calcutta University, I knelt at my guru's feet and thanked him for all the blessings flowing from his life into mine.

"Get up, Mukunda," he said indulgently. "The Lord simply found it more convenient to make you a graduate than to rearrange the sun and moon!"

[1] I must do Professor Ghoshal the justice of admitting that the strained relationship between us was not due to any fault of his, but solely to my absences from classes and inattention in them. Professor Ghoshal was, and is, a remarkable orator with vast philosophical knowledge. In later years we came to a cordial understanding.

[2] Although my cousin and I have the same family name of Ghosh, Prabhas has accustomed himself to transliterating his name in English as Ghose; therefore I follow his own spelling here.

[3] A disciple always removes his shoes in an Indian hermitage.

[4] Matthew 6:33.

## CHAPTER 24

# *I Become a Monk of the Swami Order*

"Master, my father has been anxious for me to accept an executive position with the Bengal-Nagpur Railway. But I have definitely refused it." I added hopefully, "Sir, will you not make me a monk of the Swami Order?" I looked pleadingly at my guru. During preceding years, in order to test the depth of my determination, he had refused this same request. Today, however, he smiled graciously.

"Very well; tomorrow I will initiate you into swamiship." He went on quietly, "I am happy that you have persisted in your desire to be a monk. Lahiri Mahasaya often said: 'If you don't invite God to be your summer Guest, He won't come in the winter of your life.'"

"Dear master, I could never falter in my goal to belong to the Swami Order like your revered self." I smiled at him with measureless affection.

"He that is unmarried careth for the things that belong to the Lord, how he may please the Lord: but he that is married careth for the things of the world, how he may please his wife."[1] I had analyzed the lives of many of my friends who, after undergoing certain spiritual discipline, had then married. Launched on the sea of worldly responsibilities, they had forgotten their resolutions to meditate deeply.

To allot God a secondary place in life was, to me, inconceivable. Though He is the sole Owner of the cosmos, silently showering us with gifts from life to life, one thing yet remains which He does not own, and which each human heart is empowered to withhold or bestow-man's love. The Creator, in taking infinite pains to shroud with mystery His presence in every atom of creation, could have had but one motive-a sensitive desire that men seek Him only through free will. With what velvet glove of every humility has He not covered the iron hand of omnipotence!

The following day was one of the most memorable in my life. It was a sunny Thursday, I remember, in July, 1914, a few weeks after my graduation from college. On the inner balcony of his Serampore hermitage, Master dipped a new piece of white silk into a dye of ocher, the traditional color of the Swami Order. After the cloth had dried, my guru draped it around me as a renunciate's robe.

"Someday you will go to the West, where silk is preferred," he said. "As a symbol, I have chosen for you this silk material instead of the customary cotton."

In India, where monks embrace the ideal of poverty, a silk-clad swami is an unusual sight. Many yogis, however, wear garments of silk, which preserves certain subtle bodily currents better than cotton.

"I am averse to ceremonies," Sri Yukteswar remarked. "I will make you a swami in the *bidwat* (non-ceremonious) manner."

The *bibidisa* or elaborate initiation into swamiship includes a fire ceremony, during which symbolical funeral rites are performed. The physical body of the disciple is represented as dead, cremated in the flame of wisdom. The newly-made swami is then given a chant, such as: "This *atma* is Brahma"[2] or "Thou art That" or "I am He." Sri Yukteswar, however, with his love of simplicity, dispensed with all formal rites and merely asked me to select a new name.

"I will give you the privilege of choosing it yourself," he said, smiling.

"Yogananda," I replied, after a moment's thought. The name literally means "Bliss (*ananda*) through divine union (*yoga*)."

"Be it so. Forsaking your family name of Mukunda Lal Ghosh, henceforth you shall be called Yogananda of the Giri branch of the Swami Order."

As I knelt before Sri Yukteswar, and for the first time heard him pronounce my new name, my heart overflowed with gratitude. How lovingly and tirelessly had he labored, that the boy Mukunda be someday transformed into the monk Yogananda! I joyfully sang a few verses from the long Sanskrit chant of Lord Shankara:

*"Mind, nor intellect, nor ego, feeling;*

*Sky nor earth nor metals am I.*

*I am He, I am He, Blessed Spirit, I am He!*

*No birth, no death, no caste have I;*

*Father, mother, have I none.*

*I am He, I am He, Blessed Spirit, I am He!*

*Beyond the flights of fancy, formless am I,*

*Permeating the limbs of all life;*

*Bondage I do not fear; I am free, ever free,*

*I am He, I am He, Blessed Spirit, I am He!"*

Every swami belongs to the ancient monastic order which was organized in its present form by Shankara.[3] Because it is a formal order, with an unbroken line of saintly representatives serving as active leaders, no man can give himself the title of swami. He rightfully receives it only from another swami; all monks thus trace their spiritual lineage to one common guru, Lord Shankara. By vows of poverty, chastity, and obedience to the spiritual teacher, many Catholic Christian monastic orders resemble the Order of Swamis.

In addition to his new name, usually ending in *ananda,* the swami takes a title which indicates his formal connection with one of the ten subdivisions of the Swami Order. These *dasanamis* or ten agnomens include the *Giri* (mountain), to which Sri Yukteswar, and hence myself, belong. Among the other branches are the *Sagar* (sea), *Bharati* (land), *Aranya* (forest), *Puri* (tract), *Tirtha* (place of pilgrimage), and *Saraswati* (wisdom of nature).

The new name received by a swami thus has a twofold significance, and represents the attainment of supreme bliss ( *ananda*) through some divine quality or state-love, wisdom, devotion, service, yoga-and through a harmony with nature, as expressed in her infinite vastness of oceans, mountains, skies.

The ideal of selfless service to all mankind, and of renunciation of personal ties and ambitions, leads the majority of swamis to engage actively in humanitarian and educational work in India, or occasionally in foreign lands. Ignoring all prejudices of caste, creed, class, color, sex, or race, a swami follows the precepts of human brotherhood. His goal is absolute unity with Spirit. Imbuing his waking and sleeping consciousness with the thought, "I am He," he roams contentedly, in the world but not of it. Thus only may he justify his title of swami-one who seeks to achieve union with the *Swa* or Self. It is needless to add that not all formally titled swamis are equally successful in reaching their high goal.

Sri Yukteswar was both a swami and a yogi. A swami, formally a monk by virtue of his connection with the ancient order, is not always a yogi. Anyone who practices a scientific technique of God-contact is a yogi; he may be either married or unmarried, either a worldly man or one of formal religious ties. A swami may conceivably follow only the path of dry reasoning, of cold renunciation; but a yogi engages himself in a definite, step-by-step procedure by which the body and mind are disciplined, and the soul liberated. Taking nothing for granted on emotional grounds, or by faith, a yogi practices a thoroughly tested series of exercises which were first mapped out by the early rishis. Yoga has produced, in every age of India, men who became truly free, truly Yogi-Christs.

Like any other science, yoga is applicable to people of every clime and time. The theory advanced by certain ignorant writers that yoga is "unsuitable for Westerners" is wholly false, and has lamentably prevented many sincere students from seeking its manifold blessings. Yoga is a method for restraining the natural turbulence of thoughts, which otherwise impartially prevent all men, of all lands, from glimpsing their true nature of Spirit. Yoga cannot know a barrier of East and West any more than does the healing and equitable light of the sun. So long as man possesses a mind with its restless thoughts, so long will there be a universal need for yoga or control.

The ancient rishi Patanjali defines "yoga" as "control of the fluctuations of the mind-stuff."[4] His very short and masterly expositions, the *Yoga Sutras,* form one of the six systems of Hindu philosophy.[5] In contradistinction to Western philosophies, all six Hindu systems embody not only theoretical but practical teachings. In addition to every conceivable ontological inquiry, the six systems formulate six definite disciplines aimed at the permanent removal of suffering and the attainment of timeless bliss.

The common thread linking all six systems is the declaration that no true freedom for man is possible without knowledge of the ultimate Reality. The later *Upanishads* uphold the *Yoga Sutras,* among the six systems, as containing the most efficacious methods for achieving direct perception of truth. Through the practical techniques of yoga, man leaves behind forever the barren realms of speculation and cognizes in experience the veritable Essence.

The *Yoga* system as outlined by Patanjali is known as the Eightfold Path. The first steps, (1) *yama* and (2) *niyama,* require observance of ten negative and positive moralities-avoidance of injury to others, of untruthfulness, of stealing, of incontinence, of gift-receiving (which brings obligations); and purity of body and mind, contentment, self-discipline, study, and devotion to God.

The next steps are (3) *asana* (right posture); the spinal column must be held straight, and the body firm in a comfortable position for meditation; (4) *pranayama* (control of *prana,* subtle life currents); and (5) *pratyahara* (withdrawal of the senses from external objects).

The last steps are forms of yoga proper: (6) *dharana* (concentration); holding the mind to one thought; (7) *dhyana* (meditation), and (8) *samadhi* (superconscious perception). This is the Eightfold Path of Yoga[6] which leads one to the final goal of *Kaivalya* (Absoluteness), a term which might be more comprehensibly put as "realization of the Truth beyond all intellectual apprehension."

"Which is greater," one may ask, "a swami or a yogi?" If and when final oneness with God is achieved, the distinctions of the various paths disappear. The *Bhagavad Gita,* however, points out that the methods of yoga are all-embracive. Its techniques are not meant only for certain types and temperaments, such as those few who incline toward the monastic life; yoga requires no formal allegiance. Because the yogic science satisfies a universal need, it has a natural universal applicability.

A true yogi may remain dutifully in the world; there he is like butter on water, and not like the easily-diluted milk of unchurned and undisciplined humanity. To fulfill one's earthly responsibilities is indeed the higher path, provided the yogi, maintaining a mental uninvolvement with egotistical desires, plays his part as a willing instrument of God.

There are a number of great souls, living in American or European or other non-Hindu bodies today who, though they may never have heard the words *yogi* and *swami,* are yet true exemplars of those terms. Through their disinterested service to mankind, or through their mastery over passions and thoughts, or through their single hearted love of God, or through their great powers of concentration, they are, in a sense, yogis; they have set themselves the goal of yoga-self-control. These men could rise to even greater heights if they were taught the definite science of yoga, which makes possible a more conscious direction of one's mind and life.

Yoga has been superficially misunderstood by certain Western writers, but its critics have never been its practitioners. Among many thoughtful tributes to yoga may be mentioned one by Dr. C. G. Jung, the famous Swiss psychologist.

"When a religious method recommends itself as 'scientific,' it can be certain of its public in the West. Yoga fulfills this expectation," Dr. Jung writes.[7] "Quite apart from the charm of the new, and the fascination of the half-understood, there is good cause for Yoga to have many adherents. It offers the possibility of controllable experience, and thus satisfies the scientific need of 'facts,' and besides this, by reason of its breadth and depth, its venerable age, its doctrine and method, which include every phase of life, it promises undreamed-of possibilities.

"Every religious or philosophical practice means a psychological discipline, that is, a method of mental hygiene. The manifold, purely bodily procedures of Yoga[8] also mean a physiological hygiene which is superior to ordinary gymnastics and breathing exercises, inasmuch as it is not merely mechanistic and scientific, but also philosophical; in its training of the parts of the body, it unites them with the whole of the spirit, as is quite clear, for instance, in the *Pranayama* exercises where *Prana* is both the breath and the universal dynamics of the cosmos.

"When the thing which the individual is doing is also a cosmic event, the effect experienced in the body (the innervation), unites with the emotion of the spirit (the universal idea), and out of this there develops a lively unity which no technique, however scientific, can produce. Yoga practice is unthinkable, and would also be ineffectual, without the concepts on which Yoga is based. It combines the bodily and the spiritual with each other in an extraordinarily complete way.

"In the East, where these ideas and practices have developed, and where for several thousand years an unbroken tradition has created the necessary spiritual foundations, Yoga is, as I can readily believe, the perfect and appropriate method of fusing body and mind together so that they form a unity which is scarcely to be questioned. This unity creates a psychological disposition which makes possible intuitions that transcend consciousness."

The Western day is indeed nearing when the inner science of self-control will be found as necessary as the outer conquest of nature. This new Atomic Age will see men's minds sobered and broadened by the now scientifically indisputable truth that matter is in reality a concentrate of energy. Finer forces of the human mind can and must liberate energies greater than those within stones and metals, lest the material atomic giant, newly unleashed, turn on the world in mindless destruction.[9]

[1] I Corinthians 7:32-33.

[2] Literally, "This soul is Spirit." The Supreme Spirit, the Uncreated, is wholly unconditioned (neti, neti, not this, not that) but is often referred to in Vedanta as Sat-Chit-Ananda, that is, Being-Intelligence-Bliss.

[3] Sometimes called Shankaracharya. Acharya means "religious teacher." Shankara's date is a center of the usual scholastic dispute. A few records indicate that the peerless monist lived from 510 to 478 B.C.; Western historians assign him to the late eighth century A.D. Readers who are interested in Shankara's famous exposition of the Brahma Sutras will find a careful English translation in Dr. Paul Deussen's System of the Vedanta (Chicago: Open Court Publishing Company, 1912). Short extracts from his writings will be found in Selected Works of Sri Shankaracharya (Natesan & Co., Madras).

[4] "Chitta vritti nirodha"-Yoga Sutra I:2. Patanjali's date is unknown, though a number of scholars place him in the second century B.C. The rishis gave forth treatises on all subjects with such insight that ages have been powerless to outmode them; yet, to the subsequent consternation of historians, the sages made no effort to attach their own dates and personalities to their literary works. They knew their lives were only temporarily important as flashes of the great infinite Life;

and that truth is timeless, impossible to trademark, and no private possession of their own.

[5] The six orthodox systems (saddarsana) are Sankhya, Yoga, Vedanta, Mimamsa, Nyaya, and Vaisesika. Readers of a scholarly bent will delight in the subtleties and broad scope of these ancient formulations as summarized, in English, in History of Indian Philosophy, Vol. I, by Prof. Surendranath DasGupta (Cambridge University Press, 1922).

[6] Not to be confused with the "Noble Eightfold Path" of Buddhism, a guide to man's conduct of life, as follows (1) Right Ideals, (2) Right Motive, (3) Right Speech, (4) Right Action, (5) Right Means of Livelihood, (6) Right Effort, (7) Right Remembrance (of the Self), (8) Right Realization (samadhi).

[7] Dr. Jung attended the Indian Science Congress in 1937 and received an honorary degree from the University of Calcutta.

[8] Dr. Jung is here referring to Hatha Yoga, a specialized branch of bodily postures and techniques for health and longevity. Hatha is useful, and produces spectacular physical results, but this branch of yoga is little used by yogis bent on spiritual liberation.

[9] In Plato's Timaeus story of Atlantis, he tells of the inhabitants' advanced state of scientific knowledge. The lost continent is believed to have vanished about 9500 B.C. through a cataclysm of nature; certain metaphysical writers, however, state that the Atlanteans were destroyed as a result of their misuse of atomic power. Two French writers have recently compiled a Bibliography of Atlantis, listing over 1700 historical and other references.

**CHAPTER 25**

## *Brother Ananta and Sister Nalini*

"Ananta cannot live; the sands of his karma for this life have run out."

These inexorable words reached my inner consciousness as I sat one morning in deep meditation. Shortly after I had entered the Swami Order, I paid a visit to my birthplace, Gorakhpur, as a guest of my elder brother Ananta. A sudden illness confined him to his bed; I nursed him lovingly.

The solemn inward pronouncement filled me with grief. I felt that I could not bear to remain longer in Gorakhpur, only to see my brother removed before my helpless gaze. Amidst uncomprehending criticism from my relatives, I left India on the first available boat. It cruised along Burma and the China Sea to Japan. I disembarked at Kobe, where I spent only a few days. My heart was too heavy for sightseeing.

On the return trip to India, the boat touched at Shanghai. There Dr. Misra, the ship's physician, guided me to several curio shops, where I selected various presents for Sri Yukteswar and my family and friends. For Ananta I purchased a large carved bamboo piece. No sooner had the Chinese salesman handed me the bamboo souvenir than I dropped it on the floor, crying out, "I have bought this for my dear dead brother!"

A clear realization had swept over me that his soul was just being freed in the Infinite. The souvenir was sharply and symbolically cracked by its fall; amidst sobs, I wrote on the bamboo surface: "For my beloved Ananta, now gone."

My companion, the doctor, was observing these proceedings with a sardonic smile.

"Save your tears," he remarked. "Why shed them until you are sure he is dead?"

When our boat reached Calcutta, Dr. Misra again accompanied me. My youngest brother Bishnu was waiting to greet me at the dock.

"I know Ananta has departed this life," I said to Bishnu, before he had had time to speak. "Please tell me, and the doctor here, when Ananta died."

Bishnu named the date, which was the very day that I had bought the souvenirs in Shanghai.

"Look here!" Dr. Misra ejaculated. "Don't let any word of this get around! The professors will be adding a year's study of mental telepathy to the medical course, which is already long enough!"

Father embraced me warmly as I entered our Gurpar Road home. "You have come," he said tenderly. Two large tears dropped from his eyes. Ordinarily undemonstrative, he had never before shown me these signs of affection. Outwardly the grave father, inwardly he possessed the melting heart of a mother. In all his dealings with the family, his dual parental role was distinctly manifest.

Soon after Ananta's passing, my younger sister Nalini was brought back from death's door by a divine healing. Before relating the story, I will refer to a few phases of her earlier life.

The childhood relationship between Nalini and myself had not been of the happiest nature. I was very thin; she was thinner still. Through an unconscious motive or "complex" which psychiatrists will have no difficulty in identifying, I often used to tease my sister about her cadaverous appearance. Her retorts were equally permeated with the callous frankness of extreme youth. Sometimes Mother intervened, ending the childish quarrels, temporarily, by a gentle box on my ear, as the elder ear.

Time passed; Nalini was betrothed to a young Calcutta physician, Panchanon Bose. He received a generous dowry from Father, presumably (as I remarked to Sister) to compensate the bridegroom-to-be for his fate in allying himself with a human bean-pole.

Elaborate marriage rites were celebrated in due time. On the wedding night, I joined the large and jovial group of relatives in the living room of our Calcutta home. The bridegroom was leaning on an immense gold-brocaded pillow, with Nalini at his side. A gorgeous purple silk *sari*[1] could not, alas, wholly hide her angularity. I sheltered myself behind the pillow of my new brother-in-law and grinned at him in friendly fashion. He had never seen Nalini until the day of the nuptial ceremony, when he finally learned what he was getting in the matrimonial lottery.

Feeling my sympathy, Dr. Bose pointed unobtrusively to Nalini, and whispered in my ear, "Say, what's this?"

"Why, Doctor," I replied, "it is a skeleton for your observation!"

Convulsed with mirth, my brother-in-law and I were hard put to it to maintain the proper decorum before our assembled relatives.

As the years went on, Dr. Bose endeared himself to our family, who called on him whenever illness arose. He and I became fast friends, often joking together, usually with Nalini as our target.

"It is a medical curiosity," my brother-in-law remarked to me one day. "I have tried everything on your lean sister-cod liver oil, butter, malt, honey, fish, meat, eggs, tonics. Still she fails to bulge even one-hundredth of an inch." We both chuckled.

A few days later I visited the Bose home. My errand there took only a few minutes; I was leaving, unnoticed, I thought, by Nalini. As I reached the front door, I heard her voice, cordial but commanding.

"Brother, come here. You are not going to give me the slip this time. I want to talk to you."

I mounted the stairs to her room. To my surprise, she was in tears.

"Dear brother," she said, "let us bury the old hatchet. I see that your feet are now firmly set on the spiritual path. I want to become like you in every way." She added hopefully, "You are now robust in appearance; can you help me? My husband does not come near me, and I love him so dearly! But still more I want to progress in God-realization, even if I must remain thin[2] and unattractive."

My heart was deeply touched at her plea. Our new friendship steadily progressed; one day she asked to become my disciple.

"Train me in any way you like. I put my trust in God instead of tonics." She gathered together an armful of medicines and poured them down the roof drain.

As a test of her faith, I asked her to omit from her diet all fish, meat, and eggs.

After several months, during which Nalini had strictly followed the various rules I had outlined, and had adhered to her vegetarian diet in spite of numerous difficulties, I paid her a visit.

"Sis, you have been conscientiously observing the spiritual injunctions; your reward is near." I smiled mischievously. "How plump do you want to be-as fat as our aunt who hasn't seen her feet in years?"

"No! But I long to be as stout as you are."

I replied solemnly. "By the grace of God, as I have spoken truth always, I speak truly now.[3] Through the divine blessings, your body shall verily change from today; in one month it shall have the same weight as mine."

These words from my heart found fulfillment. In thirty days, Nalini's weight equalled mine. The new roundness gave her beauty;

her husband fell deeply in love. Their marriage, begun so inauspiciously, turned out to be ideally happy.

On my return from Japan, I learned that during my absence Nalini had been stricken with typhoid fever. I rushed to her home, and was aghast to find her reduced to a mere skeleton. She was in a coma.

"Before her mind became confused by illness," my brother-in-law told me, "she often said: 'If brother Mukunda were here, I would not be faring thus.'" He added despairingly, "The other doctors and myself see no hope. Blood dysentery has set in, after her long bout with typhoid."

I began to move heaven and earth with my prayers. Engaging an Anglo-Indian nurse, who gave me full cooperation, I applied to my sister various yoga techniques of healing. The blood dysentery disappeared.

But Dr. Bose shook his head mournfully. "She simply has no more blood left to shed."

"She will recover," I replied stoutly. "In seven days her fever will be gone."

A week later I was thrilled to see Nalini open her eyes and gaze at me with loving recognition. From that day her recovery was swift. Although she regained her usual weight, she bore one sad scar of her nearly fatal illness: her legs were paralyzed. Indian and English specialists pronounced her a hopeless cripple.

The incessant war for her life which I had waged by prayer had exhausted me. I went to Serampore to ask Sri Yukteswar's help. His eyes expressed deep sympathy as I told him of Nalini's plight.

"Your sister's legs will be normal at the end of one month." He added, "Let her wear, next to her skin, a band with an unperforated two-carat pearl, held on by a clasp."

I prostrated myself at his feet with joyful relief.

"Sir, you are a master; your word of her recovery is enough But if you insist I shall immediately get her a pearl."

My guru nodded. "Yes, do that." He went on to correctly describe the physical and mental characteristics of Nalini, whom he had never seen.

"Sir," I inquired, "is this an astrological analysis? You do not know her birth day or hour."

Sri Yukteswar smiled. "There is a deeper astrology, not dependent on the testimony of calendars and clocks. Each man is a part of the Creator, or Cosmic Man; he has a heavenly body as well as one of earth. The human eye sees the physical form, but the inward eye penetrates more profoundly, even to the universal pattern of which each man is an integral and individual part."

I returned to Calcutta and purchased a pearl for Nalini. A month later, her paralyzed legs were completely healed.

Sister asked me to convey her heartfelt gratitude to my guru. He listened to her message in silence. But as I was taking my leave, he made a pregnant comment.

"Your sister has been told by many doctors that she can never bear children. Assure her that in a few years she will give birth to two daughters."

Some years later, to Nalini's joy, she bore a girl, followed in a few years by another daughter.

"Your master has blessed our home, our entire family," my sister said. "The presence of such a man is a sanctification on the whole of India. Dear brother, please tell Sri Yukteswarji that, through you, I humbly count myself as one of his *Kriya Yoga* disciples."

---

[1] The gracefully draped dress of Indian women.

[2] Because most persons in India are thin, reasonable plumpness is considered very desirable.

[3] The Hindu scriptures declare that those who habitually speak the truth will develop the power of materializing their words. What commands they utter from the heart will come true in life.

## CHAPTER 32

# *Rama is Raised From the Dead*

"Now a certain man was sick, named Lazarus. . . . When Jesus heard that, he said, This sickness is not unto death, but for the glory of God, that the Son of God might be glorified thereby."[1]

Sri Yukteswar was expounding the Christian scriptures one sunny morning on the balcony of his Serampore hermitage. Besides a few of Master's other disciples, I was present with a small group of my Ranchi students.

"In this passage Jesus calls himself the Son of God. Though he was truly united with God, his reference here has a deep impersonal significance," my guru explained. "The Son of God is the Christ or Divine Consciousness in man. No *mortal* can glorify God. The only honor that man can pay his Creator is to seek Him; man cannot glorify an Abstraction that he does not know. The 'glory' or nimbus around the head of the saints is a symbolic witness of their *capacity* to render divine homage."

Sri Yukteswar went on to read the marvelous story of Lazarus' resurrection. At its conclusion Master fell into a long silence, the sacred book open on his knee.

"I too was privileged to behold a similar miracle." My guru finally spoke with solemn unction. "Lahiri Mahasaya resurrected one of my friends from the dead."

The young lads at my side smiled with keen interest. There was enough of the boy in me, too, to enjoy not only the philosophy but, in particular, any story I could get Sri Yukteswar to relate about his wondrous experiences with his guru.

"My friend Rama and I were inseparable," Master began. "Because he was shy and reclusive, he chose to visit our guru Lahiri

Mahasaya only during the hours of midnight and dawn, when the crowd of daytime disciples was absent. As Rama's closest friend, I served as a spiritual vent through which he let out the wealth of his spiritual perceptions. I found inspiration in his ideal companionship." My guru's face softened with memories.

"Rama was suddenly put to a severe test," Sri Yukteswar continued. "He contracted the disease of Asiatic cholera. As our master never objected to the services of physicians at times of serious illness, two specialists were summoned. Amidst the frantic rush of ministering to the stricken man, I was deeply praying to Lahiri Mahasaya for help. I hurried to his home and sobbed out the story.

"The doctors are seeing Rama. He will be well.' My guru smiled jovially.

"I returned with a light heart to my friend's bedside, only to find him in a dying state.

"He cannot last more than one or two hours,' one of the physicians told me with a gesture of despair. Once more I hastened to Lahiri Mahasaya.

"The doctors are conscientious men. I am sure Rama will be well.' The master dismissed me blithely.

"At Rama's place I found both doctors gone. One had left me a note: 'We have done our best, but his case is hopeless.'

"My friend was indeed the picture of a dying man. I did not understand how Lahiri Mahasaya's words could fail to come true, yet the sight of Rama's rapidly ebbing life kept suggesting to my mind: 'All is over now.' Tossing thus on the seas of faith and apprehensive doubt, I ministered to my friend as best I could. He roused himself to cry out:

"Yukteswar, run to Master and tell him I am gone. Ask him to bless my body before its last rites.' With these words Rama sighed heavily and gave up the ghost.[2]

"I wept for an hour by his beloved form. Always a lover of quiet, now he had attained the utter stillness of death. Another disciple came in; I asked him to remain in the house until I returned. Half-dazed, I trudged back to my guru.

"How is Rama now?' Lahiri Mahasaya's face was wreathed in smiles.

"Sir, you will soon see how he is,' I blurted out emotionally. 'In a few hours you will see his body, before it is carried to the crematory grounds.' I broke down and moaned openly.

"Yukteswar, control yourself. Sit calmly and meditate.' My guru retired into *samadhi.* The afternoon and night passed in unbroken silence; I struggled unsuccessfully to regain an inner composure.

"At dawn Lahiri Mahasaya glanced at me consolingly. 'I see you are still disturbed. Why didn't you explain yesterday that you expected me to give Rama tangible aid in the form of some medicine?' The master pointed to a cup-shaped lamp containing crude castor oil. 'Fill a little bottle from the lamp; put seven drops into Rama's mouth.'

"Sir,' I remonstrated, 'he has been dead since yesterday noon. Of what use is the oil now?'

"Never mind; just do as I ask.' Lahiri Mahasaya's cheerful mood was incomprehensible; I was still in the unassuaged agony of bereavement. Pouring out a small amount of oil, I departed for Rama's house.

"I found my friend's body rigid in the death-clasp. Paying no attention to his ghastly condition, I opened his lips with my right finger and managed, with my left hand and the help of the cork, to put the oil drop by drop over his clenched teeth.

"As the seventh drop touched his cold lips, Rama shivered violently. His muscles vibrated from head to foot as he sat up wonderingly.

"I saw Lahiri Mahasaya in a blaze of light,' he cried. 'He shone like the sun. "Arise; forsake your sleep," he commanded me. "Come with Yukteswar to see me."

"I could scarcely believe my eyes when Rama dressed himself and was strong enough after that fatal sickness to walk to the home of our guru. There he prostrated himself before Lahiri Mahasaya with tears of gratitude.

"The master was beside himself with mirth. His eyes twinkled at me mischievously.

"Yukteswar,' he said, 'surely henceforth you will not fail to carry with you a bottle of castor oil! Whenever you see a corpse, just administer the oil! Why, seven drops of lamp oil must surely foil the power of Yama!"[3]

"Guruji, you are ridiculing me. I don't understand; please point out the nature of my error.'

"I told you twice that Rama would be well; yet you could not fully believe me,' Lahiri Mahasaya explained. 'I did not mean the doctors would be able to cure him; I remarked only that they were in attendance. There was no causal connection between my two statements. I didn't want to interfere with the physicians; they have to live, too.' In a voice resounding with joy, my guru added, 'Always know that the inexhaustible Paramatman[4] can heal anyone, doctor or no doctor.'

"I see my mistake,' I acknowledged remorsefully. 'I know now that your simple word is binding on the whole cosmos.'"

As Sri Yukteswar finished the awesome story, one of the spellbound listeners ventured a question that, from a child, was doubly understandable.

"Sir," he said, "why did your guru use castor oil?"

"Child, giving the oil had no meaning except that I expected something material and Lahiri Mahasaya chose the near-by oil as an objective symbol for awakening my greater faith. The master allowed Rama to die, because I had partially doubted. But the divine guru knew that inasmuch as he had said the disciple would be well, the healing must take place, even though he had to cure Rama of death, a disease usually final!"

Sri Yukteswar dismissed the little group, and motioned me to a blanket seat at his feet.

"Yogananda," he said with unusual gravity, "you have been surrounded from birth by direct disciples of Lahiri Mahasaya. The great master lived his sublime life in partial seclusion, and steadfastly refused to permit his followers to build any organization around his teachings. He made, nevertheless, a significant prediction.

"About fifty years after my passing,' he said, 'my life will be written because of a deep interest in yoga which the West will manifest. The yogic message will encircle the globe, and aid in establishing that brotherhood of man which results from direct perception of the One Father.'

"My son Yogananda," Sri Yukteswar went on, "you must do your part in spreading that message, and in writing that sacred life."

Fifty years after Lahiri Mahasaya's passing in 1895 culminated in 1945, the year of completion of this present book. I cannot but be struck by the coincidence that the year 1945 has also ushered in a new age-the era of revolutionary atomic energies. All thoughtful minds turn as never before to the urgent problems of peace and brotherhood, lest the continued use of physical force banish all men along with the problems.

Though the human race and its works disappear tracelessly by time or bomb, the sun does not falter in its course; the stars keep their invariable vigil. Cosmic law cannot be stayed or changed, and man would do well to put himself in harmony with it. If the cosmos is against might, if the sun wars not with the planets but retires at dueful time to give the stars their little sway, what avails our mailed fist? Shall any peace indeed come out of it? Not cruelty but good will arms the universal sinews; a humanity at peace will know the endless fruits of victory, sweeter to the taste than any nurtured on the soil of blood.

The effective League of Nations will be a natural, nameless league of human hearts. The broad sympathies and discerning insight needed for the healing of earthly woes cannot flow from a mere intellectual consideration of man's diversities, but from knowledge of man's sole unity-his kinship with God. Toward realization of the world's highest ideal-peace through brotherhood-may yoga, the science of personal contact with the Divine, spread in time to all men in all lands.

Though India's civilization is ancient above any other, few historians have noted that her feat of national survival is by no means an accident, but a logical incident in the devotion to eternal verities which India has offered through her best men in every generation. By sheer continuity of being, by intransitivity before the ages-can dusty scholars truly tell us how many?-India has given the worthiest answer of any people to the challenge of time.

The Biblical story[5] of Abraham's plea to the Lord that the city of Sodom be spared if ten righteous men could be found therein, and the divine reply: "I will not destroy it for ten's sake," gains new meaning in the light of India's escape from the oblivion of Babylon, Egypt and other mighty nations who were once her contemporaries. The Lord's answer clearly shows that a land lives, not by its material achievements, but in its masterpieces of man.

Let the divine words be heard again, in this twentieth century, twice dyed in blood ere half over: No nation that can produce ten men, great in the eyes of the Unbribable Judge, shall know extinction. Heeding such persuasions, India has proved herself not witless against the thousand cunnings of time. Self-realized masters in every century have hallowed her soil; modern Christlike sages, like Lahiri Mahasaya and his disciple Sri Yukteswar, rise up to proclaim that the science of yoga is more vital than any material advances to man's happiness and to a nation's longevity.

Very scanty information about the life of Lahiri Mahasaya and his universal doctrine has ever appeared in print. For three decades in India, America, and Europe, I have found a deep and sincere interest in his message of liberating yoga; a written account of the master's life, even as he foretold, is now needed in the West, where lives of the great modern yogis are little known.

Nothing but one or two small pamphlets in English has been written on the guru's life. One biography in Bengali, *Sri Sri[6] Shyama Charan Lahiri Mahasaya,* appeared in 1941. It was written by my disciple, Swami Satyananda, who for many years has been the *acharya* (spiritual preceptor) at our *Vidyalaya* in Ranchi. I have translated a few passages from his book and have incorporated them into this section devoted to Lahiri Mahasaya.

It was into a pious Brahmin family of ancient lineage that Lahiri Mahasaya was born September 30, 1828. His birthplace was the village of Ghurni in the Nadia district near Krishnagar, Bengal. He was the youngest son of Muktakashi, the second wife of the esteemed Gaur Mohan Lahiri. (His first wife, after the birth of three sons, had died during a pilgrimage.) The boy's mother passed away during his childhood; little about her is known except the revealing fact that she was an ardent devotee of Lord Shiva,[7] scripturally designated as the "King of Yogis."

The boy Lahiri, whose given name was Shyama Charan, spent his early years in the ancestral home at Nadia. At the age of three or four he was often observed sitting under the sands in the posture of a yogi, his body completely hidden except for the head.

The Lahiri estate was destroyed in the winter of 1833, when the near-by Jalangi River changed its course and disappeared into the depths of the Ganges. One of the Shiva temples founded by the Lahiris went into the river along with the family home. A devotee rescued the stone image of Lord Shiva from the swirling waters and placed it in a new temple, now well-known as the Ghurni Shiva Site.

Gaur Mohan Lahiri and his family left Nadia and became residents of Benares, where the father immediately erected a Shiva temple. He conducted his household along the lines of Vedic discipline, with regular observance of ceremonial worship, acts of charity, and scriptural study. Just and open-minded, however, he did not ignore the beneficial current of modern ideas.

The boy Lahiri took lessons in Hindi and Urdu in Benares study-groups. He attended a school conducted by Joy Narayan Ghosal, receiving instruction in Sanskrit, Bengali, French, and English. Applying himself to a close study of the *Vedas,* the young yogi listened eagerly to scriptural discussions by learned Brahmins, including a Marhatta pundit named Nag-Bhatta.

Shyama Charan was a kind, gentle, and courageous youth, beloved by all his companions. With a well-proportioned, bright, and powerful body, he excelled in swimming and in many skillful activities.

In 1846 Shyama Charan Lahiri was married to Srimati Kashi Moni, daughter of Sri Debnarayan Sanyal. A model Indian housewife, Kashi Moni cheerfully carried on her home duties and the traditional householder's obligation to serve guests and the poor. Two saintly sons, Tincouri and Ducouri, blessed the union.

At the age of 23, in 1851, Lahiri Mahasaya took the post of accountant in the Military Engineering Department of the English government. He received many promotions during the time of his service. Thus not only was he a master before God's eyes, but also a success in the little human drama where he played his given role as an office worker in the world.

As the offices of the Army Department were shifted, Lahiri Mahasaya was transferred to Gazipur, Mirjapur, Danapur, Naini Tal, Benares, and other localities. After the death of his father, Lahiri had to assume the entire responsibility of his family, for whom he bought a quiet residence in the Garudeswar Mohulla neighborhood of Benares.

It was in his thirty-third year that Lahiri Mahasaya saw fulfillment of the purpose for which he had been reincarnated on earth. The ash-hidden flame, long smouldering, received its opportunity to burst into flame. A divine decree, resting beyond the gaze of human beings, works mysteriously to bring all things into outer manifestation at the proper time. He met his great guru, Babaji, near Ranikhet, and was initiated by him into *Kriya Yoga.*

This auspicious event did not happen to him alone; it was a fortunate moment for all the human race, many of whom were later privileged to receive the soul-awakening gift of *Kriya.* The lost, or long-vanished, highest art of yoga was again being brought to light. Many spiritually thirsty men and women eventually found their way to the cool waters of *Kriya Yoga.* Just as in the Hindu legend, where Mother Ganges offers her divine draught to the parched devotee Bhagirath, so the celestial flood of *Kriya* rolled from the secret fastnesses of the Himalayas into the dusty haunts of men.

[1] John 11:1-4.

[2] A cholera victim is often rational and fully conscious right up to the moment of death.

[3] The god of death.

[4] Literally, "Supreme soul."

[5] Genesis 18:23-32.

[6] Sri, a prefix meaning "holy," is attached (generally twice or thrice) to names of great Indian teachers.

[7] One of the trinity of Godhead-Brahma, Vishnu, Shiva-whose universal work is, respectively, that of creation, preservation, and dissolution-restoration. Shiva (sometimes spelled Siva), represented in mythology as the Lord of Renunciates, appears in visions to His devotees under various

aspects, such as Mahadeva, the matted-haired Ascetic, and Nataraja, the Cosmic Dancer.

## CHAPTER 37

## *I Go to America*

"America! Surely these people are Americans!" This was my thought as a panoramic vision of Western faces passed before my inward view.

Immersed in meditation, I was sitting behind some dusty boxes in the storeroom of the Ranchi school. A private spot was difficult to find during those busy years with the youngsters!

The vision continued; a vast multitude,[1] gazing at me intently, swept actorlike across the stage of consciousness.

The storeroom door opened; as usual, one of the young lads had discovered my hiding place.

"Come here, Bimal," I cried gaily. "I have news for you: the Lord is calling me to America!"

"To America?" The boy echoed my words in a tone that implied I had said "to the moon."

"Yes! I am going forth to discover America, like Columbus. He thought he had found India; surely there is a karmic link between those two lands!"

Bimal scampered away; soon the whole school was informed by the two-legged newspaper.[2] I summoned the bewildered faculty and gave the school into its charge.

"I know you will keep Lahiri Mahasaya's yoga ideals of education ever to the fore," I said. "I shall write you frequently; God willing, someday I shall be back."

Tears stood in my eyes as I cast a last look at the little boys and the sunny acres of Ranchi. A definite epoch in my life had now closed, I knew; henceforth I would dwell in far lands. I entrained for Calcutta a few hours after my vision. The following day I received an invitation to serve as the delegate from India to an International Congress of Religious Liberals in America. It was to convene that year in Boston, under the auspices of the American Unitarian Association.

My head in a whirl, I sought out Sri Yukteswar in Serampore.

"Guruji, I have just been invited to address a religious congress in America. Shall I go?"

"All doors are open for you," Master replied simply. "It is now or never."

"But, sir," I said in dismay, "what do I know about public speaking? Seldom have I given a lecture, and never in English."

"English or no English, your words on yoga shall be heard in the West."

I laughed. "Well, dear guruji, I hardly think the Americans will learn Bengali! Please bless me with a push over the hurdles of the English language."[3]

When I broke the news of my plans to Father, he was utterly taken aback. To him America seemed incredibly remote; he feared he might never see me again.

"How can you go?" he asked sternly. "Who will finance you?" As he had affectionately borne the expenses of my education and whole life, he doubtless hoped that his question would bring my project to an embarrassing halt.

"The Lord will surely finance me." As I made this reply, I thought of the similar one I had given long ago to my brother Ananta in Agra. Without very much guile, I added, "Father, perhaps God will put it into your mind to help me."

"No, never!" He glanced at me piteously.

I was astounded, therefore, when Father handed me, the following day, a check made out for a large amount.

"I give you this money," he said, "not in my capacity as a father, but as a faithful disciple of Lahiri Mahasaya. Go then to that far Western land; spread there the creedless teachings of *Kriya Yoga.*"

I was immensely touched at the selfless spirit in which Father had been able to quickly put aside his personal desires. The just realization had come to him during the preceding night that no ordinary desire for foreign travel was motivating my voyage.

"Perhaps we shall not meet again in this life." Father, who was sixty-seven at this time, spoke sadly.

An intuitive conviction prompted me to reply, "Surely the Lord will bring us together once more."

As I went about my preparations to leave Master and my native land for the unknown shores of America, I experienced not a little trepidation. I had heard many stories about the materialistic Western atmosphere, one very different from the spiritual background of India, pervaded with the centuried aura of saints. "An Oriental teacher who will dare the Western airs," I thought, "must be hardy beyond the trials of any Himalayan cold!"

One early morning I began to pray, with an adamant determination to continue, to even die praying, until I heard the voice of God. I wanted His blessing and assurance that I would not lose myself in the fogs of modern utilitarianism. My heart was set to go to America, but even more strongly was it resolved to hear the solace of divine permission.

I prayed and prayed, muffling my sobs. No answer came. My silent petition increased in excruciating crescendo until, at noon, I had reached a zenith; my brain could no longer withstand the pressure of my agonies. If I cried once more with an increased depth of my inner passion, I felt as though my brain would split. At that moment there came a knock outside the vestibule adjoining the Gurpar

Road room in which I was sitting. Opening the door, I saw a young man in the scanty garb of a renunciate. He came in, closed the door behind him and, refusing my request to sit down, indicated with a gesture that he wished to talk to me while standing.

"He must be Babaji!" I thought, dazed, because the man before me had the features of a younger Lahiri Mahasaya.

He answered my thought. "Yes, I am Babaji." He spoke melodiously in Hindi. "Our Heavenly Father has heard your prayer. He commands me to tell you: Follow the behests of your guru and go to America. Fear not; you will be protected."

After a vibrant pause, Babaji addressed me again. "You are the one I have chosen to spread the message of *Kriya Yoga* in the West. Long ago I met your guru Yukteswar at a *Kumbha Mela;* I told him then I would send you to him for training."

I was speechless, choked with devotional awe at his presence, and deeply touched to hear from his own lips that he had guided me to Sri Yukteswar. I lay prostrate before the deathless guru. He graciously lifted me from the floor. Telling me many things about my life, he then gave me some personal instruction, and uttered a few secret prophecies.

"*Kriya Yoga,* the scientific technique of God-realization," he finally said with solemnity, "will ultimately spread in all lands, and aid in harmonizing the nations through man's personal, transcendental perception of the Infinite Father."

With a gaze of majestic power, the master electrified me by a glimpse of his cosmic consciousness. In a short while he started toward the door.

"Do not try to follow me," he said. "You will not be able to do so."

"Please, Babaji, don't go away!" I cried repeatedly. "Take me with you!"

Looking back, he replied, "Not now. Some other time."

Overcome by emotion, I disregarded his warning. As I tried to pursue him, I discovered that my feet were firmly rooted to the floor. From the door, Babaji gave me a last affectionate glance. He raised his hand by way of benediction and walked away, my eyes fixed on him longingly.

After a few minutes my feet were free. I sat down and went into a deep meditation, unceasingly thanking God not only for answering my prayer but for blessing me by a meeting with Babaji. My whole body seemed sanctified through the touch of the ancient, ever-youthful master. Long had it been my burning desire to behold him.

Until now, I have never recounted to anyone this story of my meeting with Babaji. Holding it as the most sacred of my human experiences, I have hidden it in my heart. But the thought occurred to me that readers of this autobiography may be more inclined to believe in the reality of the secluded Babaji and his world interests if I relate that I saw him with my own eyes. I have helped an artist to draw a true picture of the great Yogi-Christ of modern India; it appears in this book.

The eve of my departure for the United States found me in Sri Yukteswar's holy presence.

"Forget you were born a Hindu, and don't be an American. Take the best of them both," Master said in his calm way of wisdom. "Be your true self, a child of God. Seek and incorporate into your being the best qualities of all your brothers, scattered over the earth in various races."

Then he blessed me: "All those who come to you with faith, seeking God, will be helped. As you look at them, the spiritual current emanating from your eyes will enter into their brains and change their material habits, making them more God-conscious."

He went on, "Your lot to attract sincere souls is very good. Everywhere you go, even in a wilderness, you will find friends."

Both of his blessings have been amply demonstrated. I came alone to America, into a wilderness without a single friend, but there I found thousands ready to receive the time-tested soul-teachings.

I left India in August, 1920, on *The City of Sparta,* the first passenger boat sailing for America after the close of World War I. I had been able to book passage only after the removal, in ways fairly miraculous, of many "red-tape" difficulties concerned with the granting of my passport.

During the two-months' voyage a fellow passenger found out that I was the Indian delegate to the Boston congress.

"Swami Yogananda," he said, with the first of many quaint pronunciations by which I was later to hear my name spoken by the Americans, "please favor the passengers with a lecture next Thursday night. I think we would all benefit by a talk on 'The Battle of Life and How to Fight It.'"

Alas! I had to fight the battle of my own life, I discovered on Wednesday. Desperately trying to organize my ideas into a lecture in English, I finally abandoned all preparations; my thoughts, like a wild colt eyeing a saddle, refused any cooperation with the laws of English grammar. Fully trusting in Master's past assurances, however, I appeared before my Thursday audience in the saloon of the steamer. No eloquence rose to my lips; speechlessly I stood before the assemblage. After an endurance contest lasting ten minutes, the audience realized my predicament and began to laugh.

The situation was not funny to me at the moment; indignantly I sent a silent prayer to Master.

"You *can!* Speak!" His voice sounded instantly within my consciousness.

My thoughts fell at once into a friendly relation with the English language. Forty-five minutes later the audience was still attentive. The talk won me a number of invitations to lecture later before various groups in America.

I never could remember, afterward, a word that I had spoken. By discreet inquiry I learned from a number of passengers: "You gave an inspiring lecture in stirring and correct English." At this delightful news I humbly thanked my guru for his timely help, realizing anew that he was ever with me, setting at naught all barriers of time and space.

Once in awhile, during the remainder of the ocean trip, I experienced a few apprehensive twinges about the coming English-lecture ordeal at the Boston congress.

"Lord," I prayed, "please let my inspiration be Thyself, and not again the laughter-bombs of the audience!"

*The City of Sparta* docked near Boston in late September. On the sixth of October I addressed the congress with my maiden speech in America. It was well received; I sighed in relief. The magnanimous secretary of the American Unitarian Association wrote the following comment in a published account[4] of the congress proceedings:

"Swami Yogananda, delegate from the Brahmacharya Ashram of Ranchi, India, brought the greetings of his Association to the Congress. In fluent English and a forcible delivery he gave an address of a philosophical character on 'The Science of Religion,' which has been printed in pamphlet form for a wider distribution. Religion, he maintained, is universal and it is one. We cannot possibly universalize particular customs and convictions, but the common element in religion can be universalized, and we can ask all alike to follow and obey it."

Due to Father's generous check, I was able to remain in America after the congress was over. Four happy years were spent in humble circumstances in Boston. I gave public lectures, taught classes, and wrote a book of poems, *Songs of the Soul,* with a preface by Dr. Frederick B. Robinson, president of the College of the City of New York.[5]

Starting a transcontinental tour in the summer of 1924, I spoke before thousands in the principal cities, ending my western trip with a vacation in the beautiful Alaskan north.

With the help of large-hearted students, by the end of 1925 I had established an American headquarters on the Mount Washington Estates in Los Angeles. The building is the one I had seen years before in my vision at Kashmir. I hastened to send Sri Yukteswar pictures of these distant American activities. He replied with a postcard in Bengali, which I here translate:

11th August, 1926

Child of my heart, O Yogananda!

Seeing the photos of your school and students, what joy comes in my life I cannot express in words. I am melting in joy to see your yoga students of different cities. Beholding your methods in chant affirmations, healing vibrations, and divine healing prayers, I cannot refrain from thanking you from my heart. Seeing the gate, the winding hilly way upward, and the beautiful scenery spread out beneath the Mount Washington Estates, I yearn to behold it all with my own eyes.

Everything here is going on well. Through the grace of God, may you ever be in bliss.

SRI YUKTESWAR GIRI

Years sped by. I lectured in every part of my new land, and addressed hundreds of clubs, colleges, churches, and groups of every denomination. Tens of thousands of Americans received yoga initiation. To them all I dedicated a new book of prayer thoughts in 1929-*Whispers From Eternity,* with a preface by Amelita Galli-

Curci.[6] I give here, from the book, a poem entitled "God! God! God!", composed one night as I stood on a lecture platform:

*From the depths of slumber,*

*As I ascend the spiral stairway of wakefulness,*

*I whisper:*

*God! God! God!*

*Thou art the food, and when I break my fast*

*Of nightly separation from Thee,*

*I taste Thee, and mentally say:*

*God! God! God!*

*No matter where I go, the spotlight of my mind*

*Ever keeps turning on Thee;*

*And in the battle din of activity*

*My silent war cry is ever: God! God! God!*

*When boisterous storms of trials shriek,*

*And when worries howl at me,*

*I drown their clamor, loudly chanting:*

*God! God! God!*

*When my mind weaves dreams*

*With threads of memories,*

*Then on that magic cloth I find embossed:*

*God! God! God!*

## Master of Kriya Yoga

*Every night, in time of deepest sleep,*

*My peace dreams and calls, Joy! Joy! Joy!*

*And my joy comes singing evermore:*

*God! God! God!*

*In waking, eating, working, dreaming, sleeping,*

*Serving, meditating, chanting, divinely loving,*

*My soul constantly hums, unheard by any:*

*God! God! God!*


Sometimes-usually on the first of the month when the bills rolled in for upkeep of the Mount Washington and other Self-Realization Fellowship centers!-I thought longingly of the simple peace of India. But daily I saw a widening understanding between West and East; my soul rejoiced.

I have found the great heart of America expressed in the wondrous lines by Emma Lazarus, carved at the base of the Statue of Liberty, the "Mother of Exiles":


*From her beacon-hand*

*Glows world-wide welcome; her mild eyes command*

*The air-bridged harbor that twin cities frame.*

*"Keep, ancient lands, your storied pomp!" cries she*

*With silent lips. "Give me your tired, your poor,*

*Your huddled masses yearning to breathe free,*

*The wretched refuse of your teeming shore.*

# The Essence of Kriya Yoga

*Send these, the homeless, tempest-tost to me,*

*I lift my lamp beside the golden door.*

[1] Many of those faces I have since seen in the West, and instantly recognized.

[2] Swami Premananda, now the leader of the Self-Realization Church of All Religions in Washington, D.C., was one of the students at the Ranchi school at the time I left there for America. (He was then Brahmachari Jotin.)

[3] Sri Yukteswar and I ordinarily conversed in Bengali.

[4] New Pilgrimages of the Spirit (Boston: Beacon Press, 1921).

[5] Dr. and Mrs. Robinson visited India in 1939, and were honored guests at the Ranchi school.

[6] Mme. Galli-Curci and her husband, Homer Samuels, the pianist, have been Kriya Yoga students for twenty years. The inspiring story of the famous prima donna's years of music has been recently published (Galli-Curci's Life of Song, by C. E. LeMassena, Paebar Co., New York, 1945).

**CHAPTER 40**

# I Return to India

Gratefully I was inhaling the blessed air of India. Our boat *Rajputana* docked on August 22, 1935 in the huge harbor of Bombay. Even this, my first day off the ship, was a foretaste of the year ahead-twelve months of ceaseless activity. Friends had gathered at the dock with garlands and greetings; soon, at our suite in the Taj Mahal Hotel, there was a stream of reporters and photographers.

Bombay was a city new to me; I found it energetically modern, with many innovations from the West. Palms line the spacious boulevards; magnificent state structures vie for interest with ancient temples. Very little time was given to sight-seeing, however; I was impatient, eager to see my beloved guru and other dear ones. Consigning the Ford to a baggage car, our party was soon speeding eastward by train toward Calcutta.[1]

Our arrival at Howrah Station found such an immense crowd assembled to greet us that for awhile we were unable to dismount from the train. The young Maharaja of Kasimbazar and my brother Bishnu headed the reception committee; I was unprepared for the warmth and magnitude of our welcome.

Preceded by a line of automobiles and motorcycles, and amidst the joyous sound of drums and conch shells, Miss Bletch, Mr. Wright, and myself, flower-garlanded from head to foot, drove slowly to my father's home.

My aged parent embraced me as one returning from the dead; long we gazed on each other, speechless with joy. Brothers and sisters, uncles, aunts, and cousins, students and friends of years long past were grouped around me, not a dry eye among us. Passed now into the archives of memory, the scene of loving reunion vividly endures, unforgettable in my heart.

As for my meeting with Sri Yukteswar, words fail me; let the following description from my secretary suffice.

"Today, filled with the highest anticipations, I drove Yoganandaji from Calcutta to Serampore," Mr. Wright recorded in his travel diary. "We passed by quaint shops, one of them the favorite eating haunt of Yoganandaji during his college days, and finally entered a narrow, walled lane. A sudden left turn, and there before us towered the simple but inspiring two-story ashram, its Spanish-style balcony jutting from the upper floor. The pervasive impression was that of peaceful solitude.

"In grave humility I walked behind Yoganandaji into the courtyard within the hermitage walls. Hearts beating fast, we proceeded up some old cement steps, trod, no doubt, by myriads of truth-seekers. The tension grew keener and keener as on we strode. Before us, near the head of the stairs, quietly appeared the Great One, Swami Sri Yukteswarji, standing in the noble pose of a sage.

"My heart heaved and swelled as I felt myself blessed by the privilege of being in his sublime presence. Tears blurred my eager sight when Yoganandaji dropped to his knees, and with bowed head offered his soul's gratitude and greeting, touching with his hand his guru's feet and then, in humble obeisance, his own head. He rose then and was embraced on both sides of the bosom by Sri Yukteswarji.

"No words passed at the beginning, but the most intense feeling was expressed in the mute phrases of the soul. How their eyes sparkled and were fired with the warmth of renewed soul-union! A tender vibration surged through the quiet patio, and even the sun eluded the clouds to add a sudden blaze of glory.

"On bended knee before the master I gave my own unexpressed love and thanks, touching his feet, calloused by time and service, and receiving his blessing. I stood then and faced two beautiful deep eyes smouldering with introspection, yet radiant with joy. We entered his sitting room, whose whole side opened to the outer balcony first seen from the street. The master braced himself against a worn davenport, sitting on a covered mattress on the cement floor. Yoganandaji and I sat near the guru's feet, with orange-colored pillows to lean against and ease our positions on the straw mat.

"I tried and tried to penetrate the Bengali conversation between the two Swamijis-for English, I discovered, is null and void when they are together, although Swamiji Maharaj, as the great guru is called by others, can and often does speak it. But I perceived the saintliness of the Great One through his heart-warming smile and twinkling eyes. One quality easily discernible in his merry, serious conversation is a decided positiveness in statement-the mark of a wise man, who knows he knows, because he knows God. His great wisdom, strength of purpose, and determination are apparent in every way.

"Studying him reverently from time to time, I noted that he is of large, athletic stature, hardened by the trials and sacrifices of renunciation. His poise is majestic. A decidedly sloping forehead, as if seeking the heavens, dominates his divine countenance. He has a rather large and homely nose, with which he amuses himself in idle moments, flipping and wiggling it with his fingers, like a child. His powerful dark eyes are haloed by an ethereal blue ring. His hair, parted in the middle, begins as silver and changes to streaks of silvery-gold and silvery-black, ending in ringlets at his shoulders. His beard and moustache are scant or thinned out, yet seem to enhance his features and, like his character, are deep and light at the same time.

"He has a jovial and rollicking laugh which comes from deep in his chest, causing him to shake and quiver throughout his body-very cheerful and sincere. His face and stature are striking in their power, as are his muscular fingers. He moves with a dignified tread and erect posture.

"He was clad simply in the common *dhoti* and shirt, both once dyed a strong ocher color, but now a faded orange.

"Glancing about, I observed that this rather dilapidated room suggested the owner's non-attachment to material comforts. The weather-stained white walls of the long chamber were streaked with fading blue plaster. At one end of the room hung a picture of Lahiri Mahasaya, garlanded in simple devotion. There was also an old picture showing Yoganandaji as he had first arrived in Boston, standing with the other delegates to the Congress of Religions.

"I noted a quaint concurrence of modernity and antiquation. A huge, cut-glass, candle-light chandelier was covered with cobwebs through disuse, and on the wall was a bright, up-to-date calendar. The whole room emanated a fragrance of peace and calmness. Beyond the balcony I could see coconut trees towering over the hermitage in silent protection.

"It is interesting to observe that the master has merely to clap his hands together and, before finishing, he is served or attended by some small disciple. Incidentally, I am much attracted to one of them-a thin lad, named Prafulla,[2] with long black hair to his shoulders, a most penetrating pair of sparkling black eyes, and a heavenly smile; his eyes twinkle, as the corners of his mouth rise, like the stars and the crescent moon appearing at twilight.

"Swami Sri Yukteswarji's joy is obviously intense at the return of his 'product' (and he seems to be somewhat inquisitive about the 'product's product'). However, predominance of the wisdom-aspect in the Great One's nature hinders his outward expression of feeling.

"Yoganandaji presented him with some gifts, as is the custom when the disciple returns to his guru. We sat down later to a simple but well-cooked meal. All the dishes were vegetable and rice combinations. Sri Yukteswarji was pleased at my use of a number of Indian customs, 'finger-eating' for example.

"After several hours of flying Bengali phrases and the exchange of warm smiles and joyful glances, we paid obeisance at his feet, bade adieu with a *pronam,*[3] and departed for Calcutta with an everlasting memory of a sacred meeting and greeting. Although I write chiefly of my external impressions of him, yet I was always conscious of the true basis of the saint-his spiritual glory. I felt his power, and shall carry that feeling as my divine blessing."

From America, Europe, and Palestine I had brought many presents for Sri Yukteswar. He received them smilingly, but without remark. For my own use, I had bought in Germany a combination umbrella-cane. In India I decided to give the cane to Master.

"This gift I appreciate indeed!" My guru's eyes were turned on me with affectionate understanding as he made the unwonted comment. From all the presents, it was the cane that he singled out to display to visitors.

"Master, please permit me to get a new carpet for the sitting room." I had noticed that Sri Yukteswar's tiger skin was placed over a torn rug.

"Do so if it pleases you." My guru's voice was not enthusiastic. "Behold, my tiger mat is nice and clean; I am monarch in my own little kingdom. Beyond it is the vast world, interested only in externals."

As he uttered these words I felt the years roll back; once again I am a young disciple, purified in the daily fires of chastisement!

As soon as I could tear myself away from Serampore and Calcutta, I set out, with Mr. Wright, for Ranchi. What a welcome there, a veritable ovation! Tears stood in my eyes as I embraced the selfless teachers who had kept the banner of the school flying during my fifteen years' absence. The bright faces and happy smiles of the residential and day students were ample testimony to the worth of their many-sided school and yoga training.

Yet, alas! the Ranchi institution was in dire financial difficulties. Sir Manindra Chandra Nundy, the old Maharaja whose Kasimbazar Palace had been converted into the central school building, and who had made many princely donations was now dead. Many free, benevolent features of the school were now seriously endangered for lack of sufficient public support.

I had not spent years in America without learning some of its practical wisdom, its undaunted spirit before obstacles. For one week I remained in Ranchi, wrestling with critical problems. Then came interviews in Calcutta with prominent leaders and educators, a long talk with the young Maharaja of Kasimbazar, a financial appeal to my father, and lo! the shaky foundations of Ranchi began to be righted. Many donations including one huge check arrived in the nick of time from my American students.

Within a few months after my arrival in India, I had the joy of seeing the Ranchi school legally incorporated. My lifelong dream of a permanently endowed yoga educational center stood fulfilled. That vision had guided me in the humble beginnings in 1917 with a group of seven boys.

In the decade since 1935, Ranchi has enlarged its scope far beyond the boys' school. Widespread humanitarian activities are now carried on there in the Shyama Charan Lahiri Mahasaya Mission.

The school, or Yogoda Sat-Sanga Brahmacharya Vidyalaya, conducts outdoor classes in grammar and high school subjects. The residential students and day scholars also receive vocational training of some kind. The boys themselves regulate most of their activities through autonomous committees. Very early in my career as an educator I discovered that boys who impishly delight in outwitting a teacher will cheerfully accept disciplinary rules that are set by their fellow students. Never a model pupil myself, I had a ready sympathy for all boyish pranks and problems.

Sports and games are encouraged; the fields resound with hockey and football practice. Ranchi students often win the cup at competitive events. The outdoor gymnasium is known far and wide. Muscle recharging through will power is the *Yogoda* feature: mental direction of life energy to any part of the body. The boys are also taught *asanas* (postures), sword and *lathi* (stick) play, and jujitsu. The Yogoda Health Exhibitions at the Ranchi *Vidyalaya* have been attended by thousands.

Instruction in primary subjects is given in Hindi to the *Kols, Santals,* and *Mundas,* aboriginal tribes of the province. Classes for girls only have been organized in near-by villages.

The unique feature at Ranchi is the initiation into *Kriya Yoga.* The boys daily practice their spiritual exercises, engage in *Gita* chanting, and are taught by precept and example the virtues of simplicity, self-sacrifice, honor, and truth. Evil is pointed out to them as being that which produces misery; good as those actions which result in true happiness. Evil may be compared to poisoned honey, tempting but laden with death.

Overcoming restlessness of body and mind by concentration techniques has achieved astonishing results: it is no novelty at Ranchi to see an appealing little figure, aged nine or ten years, sitting for an hour or more in unbroken poise, the unwinking gaze directed to the spiritual eye. Often the picture of these Ranchi students has returned to my mind, as I observed collegians over the world who are hardly able to sit still through one class period.[4]

Ranchi lies 2000 feet above sea level; the climate is mild and equable. The twenty-five acre site, by a large bathing pond, includes one of the finest orchards in India-five hundred fruit trees-mango, guava, litchi, jackfruit, date. The boys grow their own vegetables, and spin at their *charkas.*

A guest house is hospitably open for Western visitors. The Ranchi library contains numerous magazines, and about a thousand volumes in English and Bengali, donations from the West and the East. There is a collection of the scriptures of the world. A well-classified museum displays archeological, geological, and anthropological exhibits; trophies, to a great extent, of my wanderings over the Lord's varied earth.

The charitable hospital and dispensary of the Lahiri Mahasaya Mission, with many outdoor branches in distant villages, have already ministered to 150,000 of India's poor. The Ranchi students are trained in first aid, and have given praiseworthy service to their province at tragic times of flood or famine.

In the orchard stands a Shiva temple, with a statue of the blessed master, Lahiri Mahasaya. Daily prayers and scripture classes are held in the garden under the mango bowers.

Branch high schools, with the residential and yoga features of Ranchi, have been opened and are now flourishing. These are the Yogoda Sat-Sanga Vidyapith (School) for Boys, at Lakshmanpur in Bihar; and the Yogoda Sat-Sanga High School and hermitage at Ejmalichak in Midnapore.

A stately Yogoda Math was dedicated in 1939 at Dakshineswar, directly on the Ganges. Only a few miles north of Calcutta, the new hermitage affords a haven of peace for city dwellers. Suitable accommodations are available for Western guests, and particularly for those seekers who are intensely dedicating their lives to spiritual realization. The activities of the Yogoda Math include a fortnightly mailing of Self-Realization Fellowship teachings to students in various parts of India.

It is needless to say that all these educational and humanitarian activities have required the self-sacrificing service and devotion of many teachers and workers. I do not list their names here, because they are so numerous; but in my heart each one has a lustrous niche. Inspired by the ideals of Lahiri Mahasaya, these teachers have abandoned promising worldly goals to serve humbly, to give greatly.

Mr. Wright formed many fast friendships with Ranchi boys; clad in a simple *dhoti,* he lived for awhile among them. At Ranchi, Calcutta, Serampore, everywhere he went, my secretary, who has a vivid gift of description, hauled out his travel diary to record his adventures. One evening I asked him a question.

"Dick, what is your impression of India?"

"Peace," he said thoughtfully. "The racial aura is peace."

---

[1] We broke our journey in Central Provinces, halfway across the continent, to see Mahatma Gandhi at Wardha. Those days are described in chapter 44.

[2] Prafulla was the lad who had been present with Master when a cobra approached (see page 116).

[3] Literally, "holy name," a word of greeting among Hindus, accompanied by palm-folded hands lifted from the heart to the forehead in salutation. A pronam in India takes the place of the Western greeting by handshaking.

[4] Mental training through certain concentration techniques has produced in each Indian generation men of prodigious memory. Sir T. Vijayaraghavachari, in the Hindustan Times, has described the tests put to the modern professional "memory men" of Madras. "These men," he wrote, "were unusually learned in Sanskrit literature. Seated in the midst of a large audience, they were equal to the tests that several members of the audience simultaneously put them to. The test would be like this: one person would start ringing a bell, the number of rings having to be counted by the 'memory man.' A second person would dictate from a paper a long exercise in arithmetic, involving addition, subtraction, multiplication, and division. A third would go on reciting from the Ramayana or the Mahabharata a long series of poems, which had to be reproduced; a fourth would set problems in versification which required the composition of verses in proper meter on a given subject, each line to end in a specified word, a fifth man would carry on with a sixth a theological disputation, the exact language of which had to be quoted in the precise order in which the disputants conducted it, and a seventh man was all the while turning a wheel, the number of revolutions of which had to be counted. The memory expert had simultaneously to do all these feats purely by mental processes, as he was allowed no paper and pencil. The strain on the faculties must have been terrific. Ordinarily men in unconscious envy are apt to depreciate such efforts by affecting to believe that they involve only the exercise of the lower functionings of the brain. It is not, however, a pure question of memory. The greater factor is the immense concentration of mind."

## CHAPTER 42

# *Last Days With My Guru*

"Guruji, I am glad to find you alone this morning." I had just arrived at the Serampore hermitage, carrying a fragrant burden of fruit and roses. Sri Yukteswar glanced at me meekly.

"What is your question?" Master looked about the room as though he were seeking escape.

"Guruji, I came to you as a high-school youth; now I am a grown man, even with a gray hair or two. Though you have showered me with silent affection from the first hour to this, do you realize that once only, on the day of meeting, have you ever said, 'I love you'?" I looked at him pleadingly.

Master lowered his gaze. "Yogananda, must I bring out into the cold realms of speech the warm sentiments best guarded by the wordless heart?"

"Guruji, I know you love me, but my mortal ears ache to hear you say so."

"Be it as you wish. During my married life I often yearned for a son, to train in the yogic path. But when you came into my life, I was content; in you I have found my son." Two clear teardrops stood in Sri Yukteswar's eyes. "Yogananda, I love you always."

"Your answer is my passport to heaven." I felt a weight lift from my heart, dissolved forever at his words. Often had I wondered at his silence. Realizing that he was unemotional and self-contained, yet sometimes I feared I had been unsuccessful in fully satisfying him. His was a strange nature, never utterly to be known; a nature deep and still, unfathomable to the outer world, whose values he had long transcended.

A few days later, when I spoke before a huge audience at Albert Hall in Calcutta, Sri Yukteswar consented to sit beside me on the platform, with the Maharaja of Santosh and the Mayor of Calcutta. Though Master made no remark to me, I glanced at him from time to time during my address, and thought I detected a pleased twinkle in his eyes.

Then came a talk before the alumni of Serampore College. As I gazed upon my old classmates, and as they gazed on their own "Mad Monk," tears of joy showed unashamedly. My silver-tongued professor of philosophy, Dr. Ghoshal, came forward to greet me, all our past misunderstandings dissolved by the alchemist Time.

A Winter Solstice Festival was celebrated at the end of December in the Serampore hermitage. As always, Sri Yukteswar's disciples gathered from far and near. Devotional *sankirtans,* solos in the nectar-sweet voice of Kristo-da, a feast served by young disciples, Master's profoundly moving discourse under the stars in the thronged courtyard of the ashram-memories, memories! Joyous festivals of years long past! Tonight, however, there was to be a new feature.

"Yogananda, please address the assemblage-in English." Master's eyes were twinkling as he made this doubly unusual request; was he thinking of the shipboard predicament that had preceded my first lecture in English? I told the story to my audience of brother disciples, ending with a fervent tribute to our guru.

"His omnipresent guidance was with me not alone on the ocean steamer," I concluded, "but daily throughout my fifteen years in the vast and hospitable land of America."

After the guests had departed, Sri Yukteswar called me to the same bedroom where-once only, after a festival of my early years-I had been permitted to sleep on his wooden bed. Tonight my guru was sitting there quietly, a semicircle of disciples at his feet. He smiled as I quickly entered the room.

"Yogananda, are you leaving now for Calcutta? Please return here tomorrow. I have certain things to tell you."

The next afternoon, with a few simple words of blessing, Sri Yukteswar bestowed on me the further monastic title of *Paramhansa.*[1]

"It now formally supersedes your former title of *swami,*" he said as I knelt before him. With a silent chuckle I thought of the struggle which my American students would undergo over the pronunciation of *Paramhansaji.*[2]

"My task on earth is now finished; you must carry on." Master spoke quietly, his eyes calm and gentle. My heart was palpitating in fear.

"Please send someone to take charge of our ashram at Puri," Sri Yukteswar went on. "I leave everything in your hands. You will be able to successfully sail the boat of your life and that of the organization to the divine shores."

In tears, I was embracing his feet; he rose and blessed me endearingly.

The following day I summoned from Ranchi a disciple, Swami Sebananda, and sent him to Puri to assume the hermitage duties.[3] Later my guru discussed with me the legal details of settling his estate; he was anxious to prevent the possibility of litigation by relatives, after his death, for possession of his two hermitages and other properties, which he wished to be deeded over solely for charitable purposes.

"Arrangements were recently made for Master to visit Kidderpore,[4] but he failed to go." Amulaya Babu, a brother disciple, made this remark to me one afternoon; I felt a cold wave of premonition. To my pressing inquiries, Sri Yukteswar only replied, "I shall go to Kidderpore no more." For a moment, Master trembled like a frightened child.

("Attachment to bodily residence, springing up of its own nature [i.e., arising from immemorial roots, past experiences of death]," Patanjali wrote,[5] "is present in slight degree even in great saints." In some of his discourses on death, my guru had been wont to add: "Just as a long-caged bird hesitates to leave its accustomed home when the door is opened.")

"Guruji," I entreated him with a sob, "don't say that! Never utter those words to me!"

Sri Yukteswar's face relaxed in a peaceful smile. Though nearing his eighty-first birthday, he looked well and strong.

Basking day by day in the sunshine of my guru's love, unspoken but keenly felt, I banished from my conscious mind the various hints he had given of his approaching passing.

"Sir, the *Kumbha Mela* is convening this month at Allahabad." I showed Master the *mela* dates in a Bengali almanac.[6]

"Do you really want to go?"

Not sensing Sri Yukteswar's reluctance to have me leave him, I went on, "Once you beheld the blessed sight of Babaji at an Allahabad *kumbha*. Perhaps this time I shall be fortunate enough to see him."

"I do not think you will meet him there." My guru then fell into silence, not wishing to obstruct my plans.

When I set out for Allahabad the following day with a small group, Master blessed me quietly in his usual manner. Apparently I was remaining oblivious to implications in Sri Yukteswar's attitude because the Lord wished to spare me the experience of being forced, helplessly, to witness my guru's passing. It has always happened in my life that, at the death of those dearly beloved by me, God has compassionately arranged that I be distant from the scene.[7]

Our party reached the *Kumbha Mela* on January 23, 1936. The surging crowd of nearly two million persons was an impressive sight, even an overwhelming one. The peculiar genius of the Indian people is the reverence innate in even the lowliest peasant for the worth of the Spirit, and for the monks and sadhus who have forsaken worldly ties to seek a diviner anchorage. Imposters and hypocrites there are indeed, but India respects all for the sake of the few who illumine the whole land with supernal blessings. Westerners who were viewing the vast spectacle had a unique opportunity to feel the pulse of the land, the spiritual ardor to which India owes her quenchless vitality before the blows of time.

The first day was spent by our group in sheer staring. Here were countless bathers, dipping in the holy river for remission of sins; there we saw solemn rituals of worship; yonder were devotional offerings being strewn at the dusty feet of saints; a turn of our heads, and a line of elephants, caparisoned horses and slow-paced Rajputana camels filed by, or a quaint religious parade of naked sadhus, waving scepters of gold and silver, or flags and streamers of silken velvet.

Anchorites wearing only loincloths sat quietly in little groups, their bodies besmeared with the ashes that protect them from the heat and cold. The spiritual eye was vividly represented on their foreheads by a single spot of sandalwood paste. Shaven-headed swamis appeared by the thousands, ocher-robed and carrying their bamboo staff and begging bowl. Their faces beamed with the renunciate's peace as they walked about or held philosophical discussions with disciples.

Here and there under the trees, around huge piles of burning logs, were picturesque sadhus,[8] their hair braided and massed in coils on top of their heads. Some wore beards several feet in length, curled and tied in a knot. They meditated quietly, or extended their hands in blessing to the passing throng-beggars, maharajas on elephants, women in multicolored *saris*- their bangles and anklets tinkling, *fakirs* with thin arms held grotesquely aloft, *brahmacharis* carrying meditation elbow-props, humble sages whose solemnity hid an inner bliss. High above the din we heard the ceaseless summons of the temple bells.

On our second *mela* day my companions and I entered various ashrams and temporary huts, offering *pronams* to saintly personages. We received the blessing of the leader of the *Giri* branch of the Swami Order-a thin, ascetical monk with eyes of smiling fire. Our next visit took us to a hermitage whose guru had observed for the past nine years the vows of silence and a strict fruitarian diet. On the central dais in the ashram hall sat a blind sadhu, Pragla Chakshu, profoundly learned in the *shastras* and highly revered by all sects.

After I had given a brief discourse in Hindi on *Vedanta,* our group left the peaceful hermitage to greet a near-by swami, Krishnananda, a handsome monk with rosy cheeks and impressive shoulders. Reclining near him was a tame lioness. Succumbing to the monk's spiritual charm-not, I am sure, to his powerful physique!-the jungle animal refuses all meat in favor of rice and milk. The swami has taught the tawny-haired beast to utter *"Aum"* in a deep, attractive growl-a cat devotee!

Our next encounter, an interview with a learned young sadhu, is well described in Mr. Wright's sparkling travel diary.

"We rode in the Ford across the very low Ganges on a creaking pontoon bridge, crawling snakelike through the crowds and over narrow, twisting lanes, passing the site on the river bank which Yoganandaji pointed out to me as the meeting place of Babaji and Sri Yukteswarji. Alighting from the car a short time later, we walked some distance through the thickening smoke of the sadhus' fires and over the slippery sands to reach a cluster of tiny, very modest mud-and-straw huts. We halted in front of one of these insignificant temporary dwellings, with a pygmy doorless entrance, the shelter of Kara Patri, a young wandering sadhu noted for his exceptional intelligence. There he sat, cross-legged on a pile of straw, his only covering-and incidentally his only possession-being an ocher cloth draped over his shoulders.

exhausted

"Truly a divine face smiled at us after we had crawled on all fours into the hut and *pronamed* at the feet of this enlightened soul, while the kerosene lantern at the entrance flickered weird, dancing shadows on the thatched walls. His face, especially his eyes and perfect teeth, beamed and glistened. Although I was puzzled by the Hindi, his expressions were very revealing; he was full of enthusiasm, love, spiritual glory. No one could be mistaken as to his greatness.

"Imagine the happy life of one unattached to the material world; free of the clothing problem; free of food craving, never begging, never touching cooked food except on alternate days, never carrying a begging bowl; free of all money entanglements, never handling money, never storing things away, always trusting in God; free of transportation worries, never riding in vehicles, but always walking on the banks of the sacred rivers; never remaining in one place longer than a week in order to avoid any growth of attachment.

"Such a modest soul! unusually learned in the *Vedas,* and possessing an M.A. degree and the title of *Shastri* (master of scriptures) from Benares University. A sublime feeling pervaded me as I sat at his feet; it all seemed to be an answer to my desire to see the real, the ancient India, for he is a true representative of this land of spiritual giants."

I questioned Kara Patri about his wandering life. "Don't you have any extra clothes for winter?"

"No, this is enough."

"Do you carry any books?"

"No, I teach from memory those people who wish to hear me."

"What else do you do?"

"I roam by the Ganges."

At these quiet words, I was overpowered by a yearning for the simplicity of his life. I remembered America, and all the responsibilities that lay on my shoulders.

"No, Yogananda," I thought, sadly for a moment, "in this life roaming by the Ganges is not for you."

After the sadhu had told me a few of his spiritual realizations, I shot an abrupt question.

"Are you giving these descriptions from scriptural lore, or from inward experience?"

"Half from book learning," he answered with a straightforward smile, "and half from experience."

We sat happily awhile in meditative silence. After we had left his sacred presence, I said to Mr. Wright, "He is a king sitting on a throne of golden straw."

We had our dinner that night on the *mela* grounds under the stars, eating from leaf plates pinned together with sticks. Dishwashings in India are reduced to a minimum!

Two more days of the fascinating *kumbha;* then northwest along the Jumna banks to Agra. Once again I gazed on the Taj Mahal; in memory Jitendra stood by my side, awed by the dream in marble. Then on to the Brindaban ashram of Swami Keshabananda.

My object in seeking out Keshabananda was connected with this book. I had never forgotten Sri Yukteswar's request that I write the life of Lahiri Mahasaya. During my stay in India I was taking every opportunity of contacting direct disciples and relatives of the Yogavatar. Recording their conversations in voluminous notes, I verified facts and dates, and collected photographs, old letters, and documents. My Lahiri Mahasaya portfolio began to swell; I realized with dismay that ahead of me lay arduous labors in authorship. I prayed that I might be equal to my role as biographer of the colossal guru. Several of his disciples feared that in a written account their master might be belittled or misinterpreted.

"One can hardly do justice in cold words to the life of a divine incarnation," Panchanon Bhattacharya had once remarked to me.

Other close disciples were similarly satisfied to keep the Yogavatar hidden in their hearts as the deathless preceptor. Nevertheless, mindful of Lahiri Mahasaya's prediction about his biography, I spared no effort to secure and substantiate the facts of his outward life.

Swami Keshabananda greeted our party warmly at Brindaban in his Katayani Peith Ashram, an imposing brick building with massive black pillars, set in a beautiful garden. He ushered us at once into a sitting room adorned with an enlargement of Lahiri Mahasaya's picture. The swami was approaching the age of ninety, but his muscular body radiated strength and health. With long hair and a snow-white beard, eyes twinkling with joy, he was a veritable patriarchal embodiment. I informed him that I wanted to mention his name in my book on India's masters.

"Please tell me about your earlier life." I smiled entreatingly; great yogis are often uncommunicative.

Keshabananda made a gesture of humility. "There is little of external moment. Practically my whole life has been spent in the Himalayan solitudes, traveling on foot from one quiet cave to another. For a while I maintained a small ashram outside Hardwar, surrounded on all sides by a grove of tall trees. It was a peaceful spot little visited by travelers, owing to the ubiquitous presence of cobras." Keshabananda chuckled. "Later a Ganges flood washed away the hermitage and cobras alike. My disciples then helped me to build this Brindaban ashram."

One of our party asked the swami how he had protected himself against the Himalayan tigers.[9]

Keshabananda shook his head. "In those high spiritual altitudes," he said, "wild beasts seldom molest the yogis. Once in the jungle I encountered a tiger face-to-face. At my sudden ejaculation, the animal was transfixed as though turned to stone." Again the swami chuckled at his memories.

"Occasionally I left my seclusion to visit my guru in Benares. He used to joke with me over my ceaseless travels in the Himalayan wilderness.

"'You have the mark of wanderlust on your foot,' he told me once. 'I am glad that the sacred Himalayas are extensive enough to engross you.'

"Many times," Keshabananda went on, "both before and after his passing, Lahiri Mahasaya has appeared bodily before me. For him no Himalayan height is inaccessible!"

Two hours later he led us to a dining patio. I sighed in silent dismay. Another fifteen-course meal! Less than a year of Indian hospitality, and I had gained fifty pounds! Yet it would have been considered the height of rudeness to refuse any of the dishes, carefully prepared for the endless banquets in my honor. In India (nowhere else, alas!) a well-padded swami is considered a delightful sight.[10]

After dinner, Keshabananda led me to a secluded nook.

"Your arrival is not unexpected," he said. "I have a message for you."

I was surprised; no one had known of my plan to visit Keshabananda.

"While roaming last year in the northern Himalayas near Badrinarayan," the swami continued, "I lost my way. Shelter appeared in a spacious cave, which was empty, though the embers of a fire glowed in a hole in the rocky floor. Wondering about the occupant of this lonely retreat, I sat near the fire, my gaze fixed on the sunlit entrance to the cave.

"'Keshabananda, I am glad you are here.' These words came from behind me. I turned, startled, and was dazzled to behold Babaji! The great guru had materialized himself in a recess of the cave. Overjoyed to see him again after many years, I prostrated myself at his holy feet.

"I called you here,' Babaji went on. 'That is why you lost your way and were led to my temporary abode in this cave. It is a long time since our last meeting; I am pleased to greet you once more.'

"The deathless master blessed me with some words of spiritual help, then added: 'I give you a message for Yogananda. He will pay you a visit on his return to India. Many matters connected with his guru and with the surviving disciples of Lahiri will keep Yogananda fully occupied. Tell him, then, that I won't see him this time, as he is eagerly hoping; but I shall see him on some other occasion.'"

I was deeply touched to receive from Keshabananda's lips this consoling promise from Babaji. A certain hurt in my heart vanished; I grieved no longer that, even as Sri Yukteswar had hinted, Babaji did not appear at the *Kumbha Mela.*

Spending one night as guests of the ashram, our party set out the following afternoon for Calcutta. Riding over a bridge of the Jumna River, we enjoyed a magnificent view of the skyline of Brindaban just as the sun set fire to the sky-a veritable furnace of Vulcan in color, reflected below us in the still waters.

The Jumna beach is hallowed by memories of the child Sri Krishna. Here he engaged with innocent sweetness in his *lilas* (plays) with the *gopis* (maids), exemplifying the supernal love which ever exists between a divine incarnation and his devotees. The life of Lord Krishna has been misunderstood by many Western commentators. Scriptural allegory is baffling to literal minds. A hilarious blunder by a translator will illustrate this point. The story concerns an inspired medieval saint, the cobbler Ravidas, who sang in the simple terms of his own trade of the spiritual glory hidden in all mankind:

*Under the vast vault of blue*

*Lives the divinity clothed in hide.*

One turns aside to hide a smile on hearing the pedestrian interpretation given to Ravidas' poem by a Western writer:

"He afterwards built a hut, set up in it an idol which he made from a hide, and applied himself to its worship."

Ravidas was a brother disciple of the great Kabir. One of Ravidas' exalted chelas was the Rani of Chitor. She invited a large number of Brahmins to a feast in honor of her teacher, but they refused to eat with a lowly cobbler. As they sat down in dignified aloofness to eat their own uncontaminated meal, lo! each Brahmin found at his side the form of Ravidas. This mass vision accomplished a widespread spiritual revival in Chitor.

In a few days our little group reached Calcutta. Eager to see Sri Yukteswar, I was disappointed to hear that he had left Serampore and was now in Puri, about three hundred miles to the south.

"Come to Puri ashram at once." This telegram was sent on March 8th by a brother disciple to Atul Chandra Roy Chowdhry, one of Master's chelas in Calcutta. News of the message reached my ears; anguished at its implications, I dropped to my knees and implored God that my guru's life be spared. As I was about to leave Father's home for the train, a divine voice spoke within.

"Do not go to Puri tonight. Thy prayer cannot he granted."

"Lord," I said, grief-stricken, "Thou dost not wish to engage with me in a 'tug of war' at Puri, where Thou wilt have to deny my incessant prayers for Master's life. Must he, then, depart for higher duties at Thy behest?"

In obedience to the inward command, I did not leave that night for Puri. The following evening I set out for the train; on the way, at seven o'clock, a black astral cloud suddenly covered the sky.[11] Later, while the train roared toward Puri, a vision of Sri Yukteswar appeared before me. He was sitting, very grave of countenance, with a light on each side.

"Is it all over?" I lifted my arms beseechingly.

He nodded, then slowly vanished.

As I stood on the Puri train platform the following morning, still hoping against hope, an unknown man approached me.

"Have you heard that your Master is gone?" He left me without another word; I never discovered who he was nor how he had known where to find me.

Stunned, I swayed against the platform wall, realizing that in diverse ways my guru was trying to convey to me the devastating news. Seething with rebellion, my soul was like a volcano. By the time I reached the Puri hermitage I was nearing collapse. The inner voice was tenderly repeating: "Collect yourself. Be calm."

I entered the ashram room where Master's body, unimaginably lifelike, was sitting in the lotus posture-a picture of health and loveliness. A short time before his passing, my guru had been slightly ill with fever, but before the day of his ascension into the Infinite, his body had become completely well. No matter how often I looked at his dear form I could not realize that its life had departed. His skin was smooth and soft; in his face was a beatific expression of tranquillity. He had consciously relinquished his body at the hour of mystic summoning.

"The Lion of Bengal is gone!" I cried in a daze.

I conducted the solemn rites on March 10th. Sri Yukteswar was buried[12] with the ancient rituals of the swamis in the garden of his Puri ashram. His disciples later arrived from far and near to honor their guru at a vernal equinox memorial service. The *Amrita Bazar Patrika,* leading newspaper of Calcutta, carried his picture and the following report:

The death *Bhandara* ceremony for Srimat Swami Sri Yukteswar Giri Maharaj, aged 81, took place at Puri on March 21. Many disciples came down to Puri for the rites.

One of the greatest expounders of the *Bhagavad Gita,* Swami Maharaj was a great disciple of Yogiraj Sri Shyama Charan Lahiri Mahasaya of Benares. Swami Maharaj was the founder of several Yogoda Sat-Sanga (Self-Realization Fellowship) centers in India, and was the great inspiration behind the yoga movement which was carried to the West by Swami Yogananda, his principal disciple. It was Sri Yukteswarji's prophetic powers and deep realization that inspired Swami Yogananda to cross the oceans and spread in America the message of the masters of India.

His interpretations of the *Bhagavad Gita* and other scriptures testify to the depth of Sri Yukteswarji's command of the philosophy, both Eastern and Western, and remain as an eye-opener for the unity between Orient and Occident. As he believed in the unity of all religious faiths, Sri Yukteswar Maharaj established *Sadhu Sabha* (Society of Saints) with the cooperation of leaders of various sects and faiths, for the inculcation of a scientific spirit in religion. At the time of his demise he nominated Swami Yogananda his successor as the president of *Sadhu Sabha.*

India is really poorer today by the passing of such a great man. May all fortunate enough to have come near him inculcate in themselves the true spirit of India's culture and *sadhana* which was personified in him.

I returned to Calcutta. Not trusting myself as yet to go to the Serampore hermitage with its sacred memories, I summoned Prafulla, Sri Yukteswar's little disciple in Serampore, and made arrangements for him to enter the Ranchi school.

"The morning you left for the Allahabad *mela,*" Prafulla told me, "Master dropped heavily on the davenport.

"Yogananda is gone!" he cried. 'Yogananda is gone!' He added cryptically, 'I shall have to tell him some other way.' He sat then for hours in silence."

My days were filled with lectures, classes, interviews, and reunions with old friends. Beneath a hollow smile and a life of ceaseless activity, a stream of black brooding polluted the inner river of bliss which for so many years had meandered under the sands of all my perceptions.

"Where has that divine sage gone?" I cried silently from the depths of a tormented spirit.

No answer came.

"It is best that Master has completed his union with the Cosmic Beloved," my mind assured me. "He is eternally glowing in the dominion of deathlessness."

"Never again may you see him in the old Serampore mansion," my heart lamented. "No longer may you bring your friends to meet him, or proudly say: 'Behold, there sits India's *Jnanavatar!*'"

Mr. Wright made arrangements for our party to sail from Bombay for the West in early June. After a fortnight in May of farewell banquets and speeches at Calcutta, Miss Bletch, Mr. Wright and myself left in the Ford for Bombay. On our arrival, the ship authorities asked us to cancel our passage, as no room could be found for the Ford, which we would need again in Europe.

"Never mind," I said gloomily to Mr. Wright. "I want to return once more to Puri." I silently added, "Let my tears once again water the grave of my guru."

[1] Literally, param, highest; hansa, swan. The hansa is represented in scriptural lore as the vehicle of Brahma, Supreme Spirit; as the symbol of discrimination, the white hansa swan is thought of as able to separate the true soma nectar from a mixture of milk and water.

[2] Ham-sa (pronounced hong-sau) are two sacred Sanskrit chant words possessing a vibratory connection with the incoming and outgoing breath. Aham-Sa is literally "I am He."

They have generally evaded the difficulty by addressing me as sir.

[3] At the Puri ashram, Swami Sebananda is still conducting a small, flourishing yoga school for boys, and meditation groups for adults. Meetings of saints and pundits convene there periodically.

[4] A section of Calcutta.

[5] Aphorisms: II:9.

[6] Religious melas are mentioned in the ancient Mahabharata. The Chinese traveler Hieuen Tsiang has left an account of a vast Kumbha Mela held in A.D. 644 at Allahabad. The largest mela is held every twelfth year; the next largest (Ardha or half) Kumbha occurs every sixth year. Smaller melas convene every third year, attracting about a million devotees. The four sacred mela cities are Allahabad, Hardwar, Nasik, and Ujjain. Early Chinese travelers have left us many striking pictures of Indian society. The Chinese priest, Fa-Hsien, wrote an account of his eleven years in India during the reign of Chandragupta II (early 4th century). The Chinese author relates: "Throughout the country no one kills any living thing, nor drinks wine. . . . They do not keep pigs or fowl; there are no dealings in cattle, no butchers' shops or distilleries. Rooms with beds and mattresses, food and clothes, are provided for resident and traveling priests without fail, and this is the same in all places. The priests occupy themselves with benevolent ministrations and with chanting liturgies; or they sit in meditation." Fa-Hsien tells us the Indian people were happy and honest; capital punishment was unknown.

[7] I was not present at the deaths of my mother, elder brother Ananta, eldest sister Roma, Master, Father, or of several close disciples.

(Father passed on at Calcutta in 1942, at the age of eighty-nine.)

[8] The hundreds of thousands of Indian sadhus are controlled by an executive committee of seven leaders, representing seven large sections of India. The present mahamandaleswar or president is Joyendra Puri. This saintly man is extremely reserved, often confining his speech to three words-Truth, Love, and Work. A sufficient conversation!

[9] There are many methods, it appears, for outwitting a tiger. An Australian explorer, Francis Birtles, has recounted that he found the Indian jungles "varied, beautiful, and safe." His safety charm was flypaper. "Every night I spread a quantity of sheets around my camp and was never disturbed," he

explained. "The reason is psychological. The tiger is an animal of great conscious dignity. He prowls around and challenges man until he comes to the flypaper; he then slinks away. No dignified tiger would dare face a human being after squatting down upon a sticky flypaper!"

[10] After I returned to America I took off sixty-five pounds.

[11] Sri Yukteswar passed at this hour-7:00 P.M., March 9, 1936.

[12] Funeral customs in India require cremation for householders; swamis and monks of other orders are not cremated, but buried. (There are occasional exceptions.) The bodies of monks are symbolically considered to have undergone cremation in the fire of wisdom at the time of taking the monastic vow.

## CHAPTER 43

# *The Resurrection of Sri Yukteswar*

"Lord Krishna!" The glorious form of the avatar appeared in a shimmering blaze as I sat in my room at the Regent Hotel in Bombay. Shining over the roof of a high building across the street, the ineffable vision had suddenly burst on my sight as I gazed out of my long open third-story window.

The divine figure waved to me, smiling and nodding in greeting. When I could not understand the exact message of Lord Krishna, he departed with a gesture of blessing. Wondrously uplifted, I felt that some spiritual event was presaged.

My Western voyage had, for the time being, been cancelled. I was scheduled for several public addresses in Bombay before leaving on a return visit to Bengal.

Sitting on my bed in the Bombay hotel at three o'clock in the afternoon of June 19, 1936-one week after the vision of Krishna-I was roused from my meditation by a beatific light. Before my open and astonished eyes, the whole room was transformed into a strange world, the sunlight transmuted into supernal splendor.

Waves of rapture engulfed me as I beheld the flesh and blood form of Sri Yukteswar!

"My son!" Master spoke tenderly, on his face an angel-bewitching smile.

For the first time in my life I did not kneel at his feet in greeting but instantly advanced to gather him hungrily in my arms. Moment of moments! The anguish of past months was toll I counted weightless against the torrential bliss now descending.

"Master mine, beloved of my heart, why did you leave me?" I was incoherent in an excess of joy. "Why did you let me go to the *Kumbha Mela?* How bitterly have I blamed myself for leaving you!"

"I did not want to interfere with your happy anticipation of seeing the pilgrimage spot where first I met Babaji. I left you only for a little while; am I not with you again?"

"But is it *you,* Master, the same Lion of God? Are you wearing a body like the one I buried beneath the cruel Puri sands?"

"Yes, my child, I am the same. This is a flesh and blood body. Though I see it as ethereal, to your sight it is physical. From the cosmic atoms I created an entirely new body, exactly like that cosmic-dream physical body which you laid beneath the dream-sands at Puri in your dream-world. I am in truth resurrected-not on earth but on an astral planet. Its inhabitants are better able than earthly humanity to meet my lofty standards. There you and your exalted loved ones shall someday come to be with me."

"Deathless guru, tell me more!"

Master gave a quick, mirthful chuckle. "Please, dear one," he said, "won't you relax your hold a little?"

"Only a little!" I had been embracing him with an octopus grip. I could detect the same faint, fragrant, natural odor which had been characteristic of his body before. The thrilling touch of his divine flesh still persists around the inner sides of my arms and in my palms whenever I recall those glorious hours.

"As prophets are sent on earth to help men work out their physical karma, so I have been directed by God to serve on an astral planet as a savior," Sri Yukteswar explained. "It is called *Hiranyaloka* or 'Illumined Astral Planet.' There I am aiding advanced beings to rid themselves of astral karma and thus attain liberation from astral rebirths. The dwellers on Hiranyaloka are highly developed spiritually; all of them had acquired, in their last earth-incarnation, the meditation-given power of consciously leaving their physical bodies at death. No one can enter Hiranyaloka unless he has passed on earth beyond the state of *sabikalpa samadhi* into the higher state of *nirbikalpa samadhi.*[1]

"The Hiranyaloka inhabitants have already passed through the ordinary astral spheres, where nearly all beings from earth must go at death; there they worked out many seeds of their past actions in the astral worlds. None but advanced beings can perform such redemptive work effectually in the astral worlds. Then, in order to free their souls more fully from the cocoon of karmic traces lodged in their astral bodies, these higher beings were drawn by cosmic law to be reborn with new astral bodies on Hiranyaloka, the astral sun or heaven, where I have resurrected to help them. There are also highly advanced beings on Hiranyaloka who have come from the superior, subtler, causal world."

My mind was now in such perfect attunement with my guru's that he was conveying his word-pictures to me partly by speech and partly by thought-transference. I was thus quickly receiving his idea-tabloids.

"You have read in the scriptures," Master went on, "that God encased the human soul successively in three bodies-the idea, or causal, body; the subtle astral body, seat of man's mental and emotional natures; and the gross physical body. On earth a man is equipped with his physical senses. An astral being works with his consciousness and feelings and a body made of lifetrons.[2] A causal-bodied being remains in the blissful realm of ideas. My work is with those astral beings who are preparing to enter the causal world."

"Adorable Master, please tell me more about the astral cosmos." Though I had slightly relaxed my embrace at Sri Yukteswar's request, my arms were still around him. Treasure beyond all treasures, my guru who had laughed at death to reach me!

"There are many astral planets, teeming with astral beings," Master began. "The inhabitants use astral planes, or masses of light, to travel from one planet to another, faster than electricity and radioactive energies.

"The astral universe, made of various subtle vibrations of light and color, is hundreds of times larger than the material cosmos. The entire physical creation hangs like a little solid basket under the huge luminous balloon of the astral sphere. Just as many physical suns and stars roam in space, so there are also countless astral solar and stellar systems. Their planets have astral suns and moons, more beautiful than the physical ones. The astral luminaries resemble the aurora borealis-the sunny astral aurora being more dazzling than the mild-rayed moon-aurora. The astral day and night are longer than those of earth.

"The astral world is infinitely beautiful, clean, pure, and orderly. There are no dead planets or barren lands. The terrestrial blemishes-weeds, bacteria, insects, snakes-are absent. Unlike the variable climates and seasons of the earth, the astral planets maintain the even temperature of an eternal spring, with occasional luminous white snow and rain of many-colored lights. Astral planets abound in opal lakes and bright seas and rainbow rivers.

"The ordinary astral universe-not the subtler astral heaven of Hiranyaloka-is peopled with millions of astral beings who have come, more or less recently, from the earth, and also with myriads of fairies, mermaids, fishes, animals, goblins, gnomes, demigods and spirits, all residing on different astral planets in accordance with karmic qualifications. Various spheric mansions or vibratory regions are provided for good and evil spirits. Good ones can travel freely, but the evil spirits are confined to limited zones. In the same way that human beings live on the surface of the earth, worms inside the soil, fish in water, and birds in air, so astral beings of different grades are assigned to suitable vibratory quarters.

"Among the fallen dark angels expelled from other worlds, friction and war take place with lifetronic bombs or mental *mantric*[3] vibratory rays. These beings dwell in the gloom-drenched regions of the lower astral cosmos, working out their evil karma.

"In the vast realms above the dark astral prison, all is shining and beautiful. The astral cosmos is more naturally attuned than the earth to the divine will and plan of perfection. Every astral object is manifested primarily by the will of God, and partially by the will-call of astral beings. They possess the power of modifying or enhancing the grace and form of anything already created by the Lord. He has given His astral children the freedom and privilege of changing or improving at will the astral cosmos. On earth a solid must be transformed into liquid or other form through natural or chemical processes, but astral solids are changed into astral liquids, gases, or energy solely and instantly by the will of the inhabitants.

"The earth is dark with warfare and murder in the sea, land, and air," my guru continued, "but the astral realms know a happy harmony and equality. Astral beings dematerialize or materialize their forms at will. Flowers or fish or animals can metamorphose themselves, for a time, into astral men. All astral beings are free to assume any form, and can easily commune together. No fixed, definite, natural law hems them round-any astral tree, for example, can be successfully asked to produce an astral mango or other desired fruit, flower, or indeed any other object. Certain karmic restrictions are present, but there are no distinctions in the astral world about desirability of various forms. Everything is vibrant with God's creative light.

"No one is born of woman; offspring are materialized by astral beings through the help of their cosmic will into specially patterned, astrally condensed forms. The recently physically disembodied being arrives in an astral family through invitation, drawn by similar mental and spiritual tendencies.

"The astral body is not subject to cold or heat or other natural conditions. The anatomy includes an astral brain, or the thousand-petaled lotus of light, and six awakened centers in the *sushumna,* or astral cerebro-spinal axis. The heart draws cosmic energy as well as light from the astral brain, and pumps it to the astral nerves and body cells, or lifetrons. Astral beings can affect their bodies by lifetronic force or by *mantric* vibrations.

"The astral body is an exact counterpart of the last physical form. Astral beings retain the same appearance which they possessed in youth in their previous earthly sojourn; occasionally an astral being chooses, like myself, to retain his old age appearance." Master, emanating the very essence of youth, chuckled merrily.

"Unlike the spacial, three-dimensional physical world cognized only by the five senses, the astral spheres are visible to the all-inclusive sixth sense-intuition," Sri Yukteswar went on. "By sheer intuitional feeling, all astral beings see, hear, smell, taste, and touch. They possess three eyes, two of which are partly closed. The third and chief astral eye, vertically placed on the forehead, is open. Astral beings have all the outer sensory organs-ears, eyes, nose, tongue, and skin-but they employ the intuitional sense to experience sensations through any part of the body; they can see through the ear, or nose, or skin. They are able to hear through the eyes or tongue, and can taste through the ears or skin, and so forth.[4]

"Man's physical body is exposed to countless dangers, and is easily hurt or maimed; the ethereal astral body may occasionally be cut or bruised but is healed at once by mere willing."

"Gurudeva, are all astral persons beautiful?"

"Beauty in the astral world is known to be a spiritual quality, and not an outward conformation," Sri Yukteswar replied. "Astral beings therefore attach little importance to facial features. They have the privilege, however, of costuming themselves at will with new, colorful, astrally materialized bodies. Just as worldly men don new array for gala events, so astral beings find occasions to bedeck themselves in specially designed forms.

"Joyous astral festivities on the higher astral planets like Hiranyaloka take place when a being is liberated from the astral world through spiritual advancement, and is therefore ready to enter the heaven of the causal world. On such occasions the

Invisible Heavenly Father, and the saints who are merged in Him, materialize Themselves into bodies of Their own choice and join the astral celebration. In order to please His beloved devotee, the Lord takes any desired form. If the devotee worshiped through devotion, he sees God as the Divine Mother. To Jesus, the Father-aspect of the Infinite One was appealing beyond other conceptions. The individuality with which the Creator has endowed each of His creatures makes every conceivable and inconceivable demand on the Lord's versatility!" My guru and I laughed happily together.

"Friends of other lives easily recognize one another in the astral world," Sri Yukteswar went on in his beautiful, flutelike voice. "Rejoicing at the immortality of friendship, they realize the indestructibility of love, often doubted at the time of the sad, delusive partings of earthly life.

"The intuition of astral beings pierces through the veil and observes human activities on earth, but man cannot view the astral world unless his sixth sense is somewhat developed. Thousands of earth-dwellers have momentarily glimpsed an astral being or an astral world.

"The advanced beings on Hiranyaloka remain mostly awake in ecstasy during the long astral day and night, helping to work out intricate problems of cosmic government and the redemption of prodigal sons, earthbound souls. When the Hiranyaloka beings sleep, they have occasional dreamlike astral visions. Their minds are usually engrossed in the conscious state of highest *nirbikalpa* bliss.

"Inhabitants in all parts of the astral worlds are still subject to mental agonies. The sensitive minds of the higher beings on planets like Hiranyaloka feel keen pain if any mistake is made in conduct or perception of truth. These advanced beings endeavor to attune their every act and thought with the perfection of spiritual law.

"Communication among the astral inhabitants is held entirely by astral telepathy and television; there is none of the confusion and misunderstanding of the written and spoken word which earth-dwellers must endure. Just as persons on the cinema screen appear to move and act through a series of light pictures, and do not actually breathe, so the astral beings walk and work as intelligently guided and coordinated images of light, without the necessity of drawing power from oxygen. Man depends upon solids, liquids, gases, and energy for sustenance; astral beings sustain themselves principally by cosmic light."

"Master mine, do astral beings eat anything?" I was drinking in his marvelous elucidations with the receptivity of all my faculties-mind, heart, soul. Superconscious perceptions of truth are permanently real and changeless, while fleeting sense experiences and impressions are never more than temporarily or relatively true, and soon lose in memory all their vividness. My guru's words were so penetratingly imprinted on the parchment of my being that at any time, by transferring my mind to the superconscious state, I can clearly relive the divine experience.

"Luminous raylike vegetables abound in the astral soils," he answered. "The astral beings consume vegetables, and drink a nectar flowing from glorious fountains of light and from astral brooks and rivers. Just as invisible images of persons on the earth can be dug out of the ether and made visible by a television apparatus, later being dismissed again into space, so the God-created, unseen astral blueprints of vegetables and plants floating in the ether are precipitated on an astral planet by the will of its inhabitants. In the same way, from the wildest fancy of these beings, whole gardens of fragrant flowers are materialized, returning later to the etheric invisibility. Although dwellers on the heavenly planets like Hiranyaloka are almost freed from any necessity of eating, still higher is the unconditioned existence of almost completely liberated souls in the causal world, who eat nothing save the manna of bliss.

"The earth-liberated astral being meets a multitude of relatives, fathers, mothers, wives, husbands, and friends, acquired during different incarnations on earth,[5] as they appear from time to time in various parts of the astral realms. He is therefore at a loss to understand whom to love especially; he learns in this way to give a divine and equal love to all, as children and individualized expressions of God. Though the outward appearance of loved ones may have changed, more or less according to the development of new qualities in the latest life of any particular soul, the astral being employs his unerring intuition to recognize all those once dear to him in other planes of existence, and to welcome them to their new astral home. Because every atom in creation is inextinguishably dowered with individuality,[6] an astral friend will be recognized no matter what costume he may don, even as on earth an actor's identity is discoverable by close observation despite any disguise.

"The span of life in the astral world is much longer than on earth. A normal advanced astral being's average life period is from five hundred to one thousand years, measured in accordance with earthly standards of time. As certain redwood trees outlive most trees by millenniums, or as some yogis live several hundred years though most men die before the age of sixty, so some astral beings live much longer than the usual span of astral existence. Visitors to the astral world dwell there for a longer or shorter period in accordance with the weight of their physical karma, which draws them back to earth within a specified time.

"The astral being does not have to contend painfully with death at the time of shedding his luminous body. Many of these beings nevertheless feel slightly nervous at the thought of dropping their astral form for the subtler causal one. The astral world is free from unwilling death, disease, and old age. These three dreads are the curse of earth, where man has allowed his consciousness to identify itself almost wholly with a frail physical body requiring constant aid from air, food, and sleep in order to exist at all.

"Physical death is attended by the disappearance of breath and the disintegration of fleshly cells. Astral death consists of the dispersement of lifetrons, those manifest units of energy which constitute the life of astral beings. At physical death a being loses his consciousness of flesh and becomes aware of his subtle body in the astral world. Experiencing astral death in due time, a being thus passes from the consciousness of astral birth and death to that of physical birth and death. These recurrent cycles of astral and physical encasement are the ineluctable destiny of all unenlightened beings. Scriptural definitions of heaven and hell sometimes stir man's deeper-than-subconscious memories of his long series of experiences in the blithesome astral and disappointing terrestrial worlds."

"Beloved Master," I asked, "will you please describe more in detail the difference between rebirth on the earth and in the astral and causal spheres?"

"Man as an individualized soul is essentially causal-bodied," my guru explained. "That body is a matrix of the thirty-five *ideas* required by God as the basic or causal thought forces from which He later formed the subtle astral body of nineteen elements and the gross physical body of sixteen elements.

"The nineteen elements of the astral body are mental, emotional, and lifetronic. The nineteen components are intelligence; ego; feeling; mind (sense-consciousness); five instruments of *knowledge*, the subtle counterparts of the senses of sight, hearing, smell, taste, touch; five instruments of *action*, the mental correspondence for the executive abilities to procreate, excrete, talk, walk, and exercise manual skill; and five instruments of *life force*, those empowered to perform the crystallizing, assimilating, eliminating, metabolizing, and circulating functions of the body. This subtle astral encasement of nineteen elements survives the death of the physical body, which is made of sixteen gross metallic and nonmetallic elements.

"God thought out different ideas within Himself and projected them into dreams. Lady Cosmic Dream thus sprang out decorated in all her colossal endless ornaments of relativity.

"In thirty-five thought categories of the causal body, God elaborated all the complexities of man's nineteen astral and sixteen physical counterparts. By condensation of vibratory forces, first subtle, then gross, He produced man's astral body and finally his physical form. According to the law of relativity, by which the Prime Simplicity has become the bewildering manifold, the causal cosmos and causal body are different from the astral cosmos and astral body; the physical cosmos and physical body are likewise characteristically at variance with the other forms of creation.

The fleshly body is made of the fixed, objectified dreams of the Creator. The dualities are ever-present on earth: disease and health, pain and pleasure, loss and gain. Human beings find limitation and resistance in three-dimensional matter. When man's desire to live is severely shaken by disease or other causes, death arrives; the heavy overcoat of the flesh is temporarily shed. The soul, however, remains encased in the astral and causal bodies.[7] The adhesive force by which all three bodies are held together is desire. The power of unfulfilled desires is the root of all man's slavery.

"Physical desires are rooted in egotism and sense pleasures. The compulsion or temptation of sensory experience is more powerful than the desire-force connected with astral attachments or causal perceptions.

"Astral desires center around enjoyment in terms of vibration. Astral beings enjoy the ethereal music of the spheres and are entranced by the sight of all creation as exhaustless expressions of changing light. The astral beings also smell, taste, and touch light. Astral desires are thus connected with an astral being's power to precipitate all objects and experiences as forms of light or as condensed thoughts or dreams.

"Causal desires are fulfilled by perception only. The nearly-free beings who are encased only in the causal body see the whole universe as realizations of the dream-ideas of God; they can materialize anything and everything in sheer thought. Causal beings therefore consider the enjoyment of physical sensations or astral delights as gross and suffocating to the soul's fine sensibilities. Causal beings work out their desires by materializing them instantly.[8] Those who find themselves covered only by the delicate veil of the causal body can bring universes into manifestation even as the Creator. Because all creation is made of the cosmic dream-texture, the soul thinly clothed in the causal has vast realizations of power.

"A soul, being invisible by nature, can be distinguished only by the presence of its body or bodies. The mere presence of a body signifies that its existence is made possible by unfulfilled desires.[9]

"So long as the soul of man is encased in one, two, or three body-containers, sealed tightly with the corks of ignorance and desires, he cannot merge with the sea of Spirit. When the gross physical receptacle is destroyed by the hammer of death, the other two coverings-astral and causal-still remain to prevent the soul from consciously joining the Omnipresent Life. When desirelessness is attained through wisdom, its power disintegrates the two remaining vessels. The tiny human soul emerges, free at last; it is one with the Measureless Amplitude."

I asked my divine guru to shed further light on the high and mysterious causal world.

"The causal world is indescribably subtle," he replied. "In order to understand it, one would have to possess such tremendous powers of concentration that he could close his eyes and visualize the astral cosmos and the physical cosmos in all their vastness-the luminous balloon with the solid basket-as existing in ideas only. If by this superhuman concentration one succeeded in converting or resolving the two cosmoses with all their complexities into sheer ideas, he would then reach the causal world and stand on the borderline of fusion between mind and matter. There one perceives all created things-solids, liquids, gases, electricity, energy, all beings, gods, men, animals, plants, bacteria-as forms of consciousness, just as a man can close his eyes and realize that he exists, even though his body is invisible to his physical eyes and is present only as an idea.

"Whatever a human being can do in fancy, a causal being can do in reality. The most colossal imaginative human intelligence is able, in mind only, to range from one extreme of thought to another, to skip mentally from planet to planet, or tumble endlessly down a pit of eternity, or soar rocketlike into the galaxied canopy, or scintillate like a searchlight over milky ways and the starry spaces. But beings in the causal world have a much greater freedom, and can effortlessly manifest their thoughts into instant objectivity, without any material or astral obstruction or karmic limitation.

"Causal beings realize that the physical cosmos is not primarily constructed of electrons, nor is the astral cosmos basically composed of lifetrons-both in reality are created from the minutest particles of God-thought, chopped and divided by *maya,* the law of relativity which intervenes to apparently separate the Noumenon from His phenomena.

"Souls in the causal world recognize one another as individualized points of joyous Spirit; their thought-things are the only objects which surround them. Causal beings see the difference between their bodies and thoughts to be merely ideas. As a man, closing his eyes, can visualize a dazzling white light or a faint blue haze, so causal beings by thought alone are able to see, hear, feel, taste, and touch; they create anything, or dissolve it, by the power of cosmic mind.

"Both death and rebirth in the causal world are in thought. Causal-bodied beings feast only on the ambrosia of eternally new knowledge. They drink from the springs of peace, roam on the trackless soil of perceptions, swim in the ocean-endlessness of bliss. Lo! see their bright thought-bodies zoom past trillions of Spirit-created planets, fresh bubbles of universes, wisdom-stars, spectral dreams of golden nebulae, all over the skiey blue bosom of Infinity!

"Many beings remain for thousands of years in the causal cosmos. By deeper ecstasies the freed soul then withdraws itself from the little causal body and puts on the vastness of the causal cosmos. All the separate eddies of ideas, particularized waves of power, love, will, joy, peace, intuition, calmness, self-control, and concentration melt into the ever-joyous Sea of Bliss. No longer does the soul have to experience its joy as an individualized wave of consciousness, but is merged in the One Cosmic Ocean, with all its waves-eternal laughter, thrills, throbs.

"When a soul is out of the cocoon of the three bodies it escapes forever from the law of relativity and becomes the ineffable Ever-Existent.[10] Behold the butterfly of Omnipresence, its wings etched with stars and moons and suns! The soul expanded into Spirit remains alone in the region of lightless light, darkless dark, thoughtless thought, intoxicated with its ecstasy of joy in God's dream of cosmic creation."

"A free soul!" I ejaculated in awe.

"When a soul finally gets out of the three jars of bodily delusions," Master continued, "it becomes one with the Infinite without any loss of individuality. Christ had won this final freedom even before he was born as Jesus. In three stages of his past, symbolized in his earth-life as the three days of his experience of death and resurrection, he had attained the power to fully arise in Spirit.

"The undeveloped man must undergo countless earthly and astral and causal incarnations in order to emerge from his three bodies. A master who achieves this final freedom may elect to return to earth as a prophet to bring other human beings back to God, or like myself he may choose to reside in the astral cosmos. There a savior assumes some of the burden of the inhabitants' karma[11] and thus helps them to terminate their cycle of reincarnation in the astral cosmos and go on permanently to the causal spheres. Or a freed soul may enter the causal world to aid its beings to shorten their span in the causal body and thus attain the Absolute Freedom."

"Resurrected One, I want to know more about the karma which forces souls to return to the three worlds." I could listen forever, I thought, to my omniscient Master. Never in his earth-life had I been able at one time to assimilate so much of his wisdom. Now for the first time I was receiving a clear, definite insight into the enigmatic interspaces on the checkerboard of life and death.

"The physical karma or desires of man must be completely worked out before his permanent stay in astral worlds becomes possible," my guru elucidated in his thrilling voice. "Two kinds of beings live in the astral spheres. Those who still have earthly karma to dispose of and who must therefore reinhabit a gross physical body in order to pay their karmic debts could be classified, after physical death, as temporary visitors to the astral world rather than as permanent residents.

"Beings with unredeemed earthly karma are not permitted after astral death to go to the high causal sphere of cosmic ideas, but must shuttle to and fro from the physical and astral worlds only, conscious successively of their physical body of sixteen gross elements, and of their astral body of nineteen subtle elements. After each loss of his physical body, however, an undeveloped being from the earth remains for the most part in the deep stupor of the death-sleep and is hardly conscious of the beautiful astral sphere. After the astral rest, such a man returns to the material plane for further lessons, gradually accustoming himself, through repeated journeys, to the worlds of subtle astral texture.

"Normal or long-established residents of the astral universe, on the other hand, are those who, freed forever from all material longings, need return no more to the gross vibrations of earth. Such beings have only astral and causal karma to work out. At astral death these beings pass to the infinitely finer and more delicate causal world. Shedding the thought-form of the causal body at the end of a certain span, determined by cosmic law, these advanced beings then return to Hiranyaloka or a similar high astral planet, reborn in a new astral body to work out their unredeemed astral karma.

"My son, you may now comprehend more fully that I am resurrected by divine decree," Sri Yukteswar continued, "as a savior of astrally reincarnating souls coming back from the causal sphere, in particular, rather than of those astral beings who are coming up from the earth. Those from the earth, if they still retain vestiges of material karma, do not rise to the very high astral planets like Hiranyaloka.

"Just as most people on earth have not learned through meditation-acquired vision to appreciate the superior joys and advantages of astral life and thus, after death, desire to return to the limited, imperfect pleasures of earth, so many astral beings, during the normal disintegration of their astral bodies, fail to picture the advanced state of spiritual joy in the causal world and, dwelling on thoughts of the more gross and gaudy astral happiness, yearn to revisit the astral paradise. Heavy astral karma must be redeemed by such beings before they can achieve after astral death a permanent stay in the causal thought-world, so thinly partitioned from the Creator.

"Only when a being has no further desires for experiences in the pleasing-to-the-eye astral cosmos, and cannot be tempted to go back there, does he remain in the causal world. Completing there the work of redeeming all causal karma or seeds of past desires, the confined soul thrusts out the last of the three corks of ignorance and, emerging from the final jar of the causal body, commingles with the Eternal.

"Now do you understand?" Master smiled so enchantingly!

"Yes, through your grace. I am speechless with joy and gratitude."

Never from song or story had I ever received such inspiring knowledge. Though the Hindu scriptures refer to the causal and astral worlds and to man's three bodies, how remote and meaningless those pages compared with the warm authenticity of my resurrected Master! For him indeed existed not a single "undiscover'd country from whose bourn no traveler returns"!

"The interpenetration of man's three bodies is expressed in many ways through his threefold nature," my great guru went on. "In the wakeful state on earth a human being is conscious more or less of his three vehicles. When he is sensuously intent on tasting, smelling, touching, listening, or seeing, he is working principally through his physical body. Visualizing or willing, he is working mainly through his astral body. His causal medium finds expression when man is thinking or diving deep in introspection or meditation;

the cosmical thoughts of genius come to the man who habitually contacts his causal body. In this sense an individual may be classified broadly as 'a material man,' 'an energetic man,' or 'an intellectual man.'

"A man identifies himself about sixteen hours daily with his physical vehicle. Then he sleeps; if he dreams, he remains in his astral body, effortlessly creating any object even as do the astral beings. If man's sleep be deep and dreamless, for several hours he is able to transfer his consciousness, or sense of I-ness, to the causal body; such sleep is revivifying. A dreamer is contacting his astral and not his causal body; his sleep is not fully refreshing."

I had been lovingly observing Sri Yukteswar while he gave his wondrous exposition.

"Angelic guru," I said, "your body looks exactly as it did when last I wept over it in the Puri ashram."

"O yes, my new body is a perfect copy of the old one. I materialize or dematerialize this form any time at will, much more frequently than I did while on earth. By quick dematerialization, I now travel instantly by light express from planet to planet or, indeed, from astral to causal or to physical cosmos." My divine guru smiled. "Though you move about so fast these days, I had no difficulty in finding you at Bombay!"

"O Master, I was grieving so deeply about your death!"

"Ah, wherein did I die? Isn't there some contradiction?" Sri Yukteswar's eyes were twinkling with love and amusement.

"You were only dreaming on earth; on that earth you saw my dream-body," he went on. "Later you buried that dream-image. Now my finer fleshly body-which you behold and are even now embracing rather closely!-is resurrected on another finer dream-planet of God. Someday that finer dream-body and finer dream-planet will pass away; they too are not forever. All dream-bubbles must eventually burst at a final wakeful touch. Differentiate, my son Yogananda, between dreams and Reality!"

This idea of *Vedantic*[12] resurrection struck me with wonder. I was ashamed that I had pitied Master when I had seen his lifeless body at Puri. I comprehended at last that my guru had always been fully awake in God, perceiving his own life and passing on earth, and his present resurrection, as nothing more than relativities of divine ideas in the cosmic dream.

"I have now told you, Yogananda, the truths of my life, death, and resurrection. Grieve not for me; rather broadcast everywhere the story of my resurrection from the God-dreamed earth of men to another God-dreamed planet of astrally garbed souls! New hope will be infused into the hearts of misery-mad, death-fearing dreamers of the world."

"Yes, Master!" How willingly would I share with others my joy at his resurrection!

"On earth my standards were uncomfortably high, unsuited to the natures of most men. Often I scolded you more than I should have. You passed my test; your love shone through the clouds of all reprimands." He added tenderly, "I have also come today to tell you: Never again shall I wear the stern gaze of censure. I shall scold you no more."

How much I had missed the chastisements of my great guru! Each one had been a guardian angel of protection.

"Dearest Master! Rebuke me a million times-do scold me now!"

"I shall chide you no more." His divine voice was grave, yet with an undercurrent of laughter. "You and I shall smile together, so long as our two forms appear different in the *maya*-dream of God. Finally we shall merge as one in the Cosmic Beloved; our smiles shall be His smile, our unified song of joy vibrating throughout eternity to be broadcast to God-tuned souls!"

Sri Yukteswar gave me light on certain matters which I cannot reveal here. During the two hours that he spent with me in the Bombay hotel room he answered my every question. A number of world prophecies uttered by him that June day in 1936 have already come to pass.

"I leave you now, beloved one!" At these words I felt Master melting away within my encircling arms.

"My child," his voice rang out, vibrating into my very soul-firmament, "whenever you enter the door of *nirbikalpa samadhi* and call on me, I shall come to you in flesh and blood, even as today."

With this celestial promise Sri Yukteswar vanished from my sight. A cloud-voice repeated in musical thunder: "Tell all! Whosoever knows by *nirbikalpa* realization that your earth is a dream of God can come to the finer dream-created planet of Hiranyaloka, and there find me resurrected in a body exactly like my earthly one. Yogananda, tell all!"

Gone was the sorrow of parting. The pity and grief for his death, long robber of my peace, now fled in stark shame. Bliss poured forth like a fountain through endless, newly opened soul-pores. Anciently clogged with disuse, they now widened in purity at the driving flood of ecstasy. Subconscious thoughts and feelings of my past incarnations shed their karmic taints, lustrously renewed by Sri Yukteswar's divine visit.

In this chapter of my autobiography I have obeyed my guru's behest and spread the glad tiding, though it confound once more an incurious generation. Groveling, man knows well; despair is seldom alien; yet these are perversities, no part of man's true lot. The day he wills, he is set on the path to freedom. Too long has he hearkened to the dank pessimism of his "dust-thou-art" counselors, heedless of the unconquerable soul.

I was not the only one privileged to behold the Resurrected Guru.

One of Sri Yukteswar's chelas was an aged woman, affectionately known as *Ma* (Mother), whose home was close to the Puri hermitage. Master had often stopped to chat with her during his morning walk. On the evening of March 16, 1936, Ma arrived at the ashram and asked to see her guru.

"Why, Master died a week ago!" Swami Sebananda, now in charge of the Puri hermitage, looked at her sadly.

"That's impossible!" She smiled a little. "Perhaps you are just trying to protect the guru from insistent visitors?"

"No." Sebananda recounted details of the burial. "Come," he said, "I will take you to the front garden to Sri Yukteswarji's grave."

Ma shook her head. "There is no grave for him! This morning at ten o'clock he passed in his usual walk before my door! I talked to him for several minutes in the bright outdoors.

"'Come this evening to the ashram,' he said.

"I am here! Blessings pour on this old gray head! The deathless guru wanted me to understand in what transcendent body he had visited me this morning!"

The astounded Sebananda knelt before her.

"Ma," he said, "what a weight of grief you lift from my heart! He is risen!"

---

[1] In sabikalpa samadhi the devotee has spiritually progressed to a state of inward divine union, but cannot maintain his cosmic consciousness except in the immobile trance-state. By continuous meditation, he reaches the superior state of nirbikalpa samadhi, where he moves freely in the world and performs his outward duties without any loss of God-realization.

[2] Sri Yukteswar used the word prana; I have translated it as lifetrons. The Hindu scriptures refer not only to the anu, "atom," and to the paramanu, "beyond the atom," finer electronic energies; but also to prana, "creative lifetronic force." Atoms and electrons are blind forces; prana is inherently intelligent. The pranic lifetrons in the spermatozoa and ova, for instance, guide the embryonic development according to a karmic design.

[3] Adjective of mantra, chanted seed-sounds discharged by the mental gun of concentration. The Puranas (ancient shastras or treatises) describe these mantric wars between devas and asuras (gods and demons). An asura once tried to slay a deva with a potent chant. But due to mispronunciation the mental bomb acted as a boomerang and killed the demon.

[4] Examples of such powers are not wanting even on earth, as in the case of Helen Keller and other rare beings.

[5] Lord Buddha was once asked why a man should love all persons equally. "Because," the great teacher replied, "in the very numerous and varied lifespans of each man, every other being has at one time or another been dear to him."

[6] The eight elemental qualities which enter into all created life, from atom to man, are earth, water, fire, air, ether, motion, mind, and individuality. (Bhagavad Gita: VII:4.)

[7] Body signifies any soul-encasement, whether gross or subtle. The three bodies are cages for the Bird of Paradise.

[8] Even as Babaji helped Lahiri Mahasaya to rid himself of a subconscious desire from some past life for a palace, as described in chapter 34.

[9] "And he said unto them, Wheresoever the body is, thither will the eagles be gathered together."-Luke 17:37. Wherever the soul is encased in the physical body or in the astral body or in the causal body, there the eagles of desires-which prey on human sense weaknesses, or on astral and causal attachments-will also gather to keep the soul a prisoner.

[10] "Him that overcometh will I make a pillar in the temple of my God, and he shall go no more out (i.e., shall reincarnate no more). . . . To him that overcometh will I grant to sit with me in my throne, even as I also overcame, and am set down with my Father in his throne."-Revelation 3:12, 21.

[11] Sri Yukteswar was signifying that, even as in his earthly incarnation he had occasionally assumed the weight of disease to lighten his disciples' karma, so in the astral world his mission as a savior enabled him to take on certain astral karma of dwellers on Hiranyaloka, and thus hasten their evolution into the higher causal world.

[12] Life and death as relativities of thought only. Vedanta points out that God is the only Reality; all creation or separate existence is maya or illusion. This philosophy of monism received its highest expression in the Upanishad commentaries of Shankara.

# Healthy Diet

## Fasting
## Magnetic Diet

## Food and Health Recipes

Selected Excerpts from Lessons and Articles

from the 1920's

FASTING

Most diseases can be cured by judicious fasting under the guidance of a specialist.

Fasting may be divided into two main groups: partial fasting and complete fasting.

*Partial Fasting*: In this group, four general subdivisions may be mentioned:

| | |
|---|---|
| (I) | Limiting the diet to certain foods; |
| (II) | Abstaining from certain foods; |
| (III) | Limiting the food intake as to quantity; |
| (IV) | Limiting the number of meals to one or two per day. |

Some of these forms of fasting may be combined. For instance, to cure disease or reduce weight, a person may abstain from certain foods altogether and limit the intake of other foods, etc.

More specific subdivisions are:

*Liquid diet*: (a) "Liquid" fasting. For one or two days a week, and whenever one does not feel hungry, the food intake may be confined to (1) milk, or (2) orange juice or any other fruit juice.

*Solid diet:* (b) "Solid" fasting. This diet is confined to (1) raw fruits; (2) raw vegetables; (3) half-boiled vegetables, including juice in which they were boiled. Drink plenty of water while on this diet.

*Oxygen diet:* (c) "Oxygen" fasting. Inhaling and exhaling deeply from six to twelve times every hour, filling the lungs with fresh air down to the lower lobes. This method may be practiced outdoors for twelve hours, while alternately slowly walking and resting. When weather conditions necessitate indoor practice, the windows should be kept wide open. (Of course, warm clothing should be worn during the winter season as a protection against the cold.) This fast aids spiritual growth. It should not be undertaken by weak individuals or invalids.

*Complete Fasting*:     Complete fasting should not, as a rule, exceed ten days and should not be attempted even for that length of time except under the supervision of a specialist. However, abstaining from food for one day each week and for three consecutive days each month has brought beneficial results. Water must be taken in abundance during complete fasting, to replace the fluid lost by evaporation through the pores, etc.

*Nine-day diet*: The Nine-day Cleansing and Vitalizing Diet, given below, has proved a most effective method for ridding the system of poisons.
>           1 ½ grapefruit
>           1 glass orange juice with tsp. Senna leaves
>           1 ½ lemons, 5 oranges
>           1 cooked vegetable with juice (quantity optional)
>           3 cups vitality beverage (one at each meal)
>           1 raw vegetable salad

*Vitality Beverage*:     Ingredients for beverage:
>           2 stalks chopped celery
>           ½ qt. chopped dandelion or turnip greens or spinach
>           5 carrots (chopped) incl. part of stem
>           1 bunch chopped parsley
>           1 qt. water
>           *No salt or spices*

The beverage may be prepared in two ways, the first being preferable:
>     (1)     After putting celery and carrots through meat chopper, lightly boil them in the water for ten minutes. Then add selected greens and parsley and boil ten minutes more. Strain by squeezing through cheesecloth.

(2)     Use the same ingredients, but do not cook them. After putting them through meat chopper, strain as above. Drink one cup of the beverage, prepared by either method, at each of the three meals.

(3)     This vitality beverage has been found to be a blood tonic and very effective in rheumatism, various stomach disorders (including acute indigestion), chronic catarrh, bronchitis, and nervous "breakdown."

While on the cleansing diet, strictly abstain from spices, candies, pastries, meat, eggs, fish, cheese, milk, butter, bread, fried foods, oil, beans – in fact, all other foods not mentioned above. If one feels the need of additional nourishment, one may take a tablespoonful of thoroughly ground nuts in a half glass of water or a glass of orange juice.

Following the nine-day diet, one should be especially careful in the selection and quantity of one's food intake the first day and resume a normal diet gradually.

If one is not successful in ridding the body of all poisons during the initial attempt, the cleansing diet may be repeated after an interval of two or three weeks.

While on the cleansing diet, it has been found beneficial every night just before going to bed, to use two pounds of some good bath salts in one-fourth tub of warm water; and also very helpful to take a bath salts bath every now and then, for several weeks after finishing the cleansing diet.

*Reducing diet:* Eat mostly raw vegetables and one-half of a boiled yolk of an egg a day. Abstain from starchy food, fried foods, and sweets. Do not drink water with meals. Every three days, fast one day on orange juice. Exercise every day.

Extremely stout people have derived much benefit from *fasting on orange juice seven days and then going on the nine-day cleansing diet, a normal diet being resumed gradually thereafter. If there was need for further reduction of weight, this procedure was repeated after an interval of two weeks.*

*Fattening Diet:* The following foods are of high nutritive value and have been found beneficial for those who wish to gain weight;

    Bananas with cream
    2 eggs
    Oatmeal with cream
    1 large raw vegetable salad
    ¼ glass cream
    1 tbsp olive oil
    2 slices whole-wheat bread
    3 ½ oz. butter

Weight has also been gained by eating bananas in abundance, and for one month drinking two glasses of water (moderately hot or cold, not iced) with each meal.

Some of the foods from the above list are added to the usual dietary.

*General dietary rules*: To have faith in God's healing power through the mind and obey dietary laws, is better than just to have faith in God and mind and disregard dietary laws.

Every day, for beneficial results, eat green-leafed vegetables, including a carrot with part of its stem, and drink a glass of orange juice (including pulp) with a tablespoonful of finely ground nuts. Mix good salad dressings made of thoroughly ground nuts, cream, a few drops of lemon juice, orange juice and honey with all salads. Thousand-island dressing is good. A little curry sauce with boiled egg or vegetables, once in a while, is a good salivary stimulant.

*Food combinations*:   For best results one should abstain from all beef and pork products. Do not make a habit of eating even chicken, lamb, or fish every day. Once a week or better, once a month is enough, if your system demands flesh foods at all. Nuts, cottage cheese, eggs, milk, cream, and bananas are very good meat and fish substitutes. If you eat chicken, lamb or fish, have a vegetable salad with them.

*Fruit should be eaten with bread or some other starchy food, but without sugar; you may add a little honey if you wish. Eat only nature's candies (unsulphured figs, prunes or raisins).*

Do not eat too much white sugar. The ingestion of excessive quantities of sweets causes intestinal fermentation.

Remember, foods prepared from white flour, such as white bread, white-flour gravy, etc., also polished rice and too many greasy fried foods, are injurious to your health.

Try to include in your daily diet as much raw food as possible. Cooked vegetables should be eaten with the juice in which they were boiled.

Catarrah of the alimentary canal often results from over-eating at night, also from eating excessively of candy or other foodstuffs which have an irritating effect on the mucous membranes of the stomach, duodenum, etc.

Fast regularly, using your best judgement as to proper diet, in accordance with the instructions given above. Eat less, and follow dietary rules when you eat. Make sunshine, oxygen, and energy a part of your regular daily diet.

*The daily diet:* Your daily food intake should be chosen from the following list of foods which contain all the elements needed for the proper maintenance of the body:

> ½ apple
> 1 baked, or half-boiled or steamed vegetable with its juice
> ¼ grapefruit
> 1 lemon

1 lime
1 raw carrot, including part of green top
1 orange
1 glass orange juice with tbsp. finely ground nuts
6 leaves raw spinach
¼ heart lettuce
1 small piece fresh pine-apple
1 tsp. olive oil
1 glass milk
6 figs, dates, or prunes
1/8 glass cream
1 handful raisins
1 tbsp. cottage cheese
1 tsp honey

Eat at least some of the above foods every day, distributing them over your three meals. For instance, you may take the milk at breakfast, bread and egg and vegetable salad at noon, and the ground nuts and fruits as night.

Individual food habits may be taken into consideration, but if they are bad, gradually change them. At any rate, add some of the foods in the above list to what you are used to eating. Omit those foods mentioned above which do not agree with you, eating only very lightly when you feel the need of nourishment, and gradually accustoming yourself to a more wholesome diet.
You may increase or decrease the quantities given above, in accordance with your individual needs. It is, of course, obvious that the person doing strenuous muscular work requires more food than the sedentary worker.

Whenever one is hungry one may take a large tablespoonful of thoroughly ground nuts in half a glass of water or in a glass of orange juice. When thirsty, drink a glass of orange juice or water (preferably distilled or boiled). However, nature's distilled water – undiluted fruit juice – is best. Do not drink too much ice water with meals. Ice water should be taken sparingly at any time, but especially during and after meals as it lowers the temperature of the stomach, thus retarding digestion. *Never drink ice water when you are overheated.*

THE MAGNETIC DIET

What distilled water is to a wet battery, food is to the body battery. The life energy in the body battery is derived from Cosmic Energy through the medulla, and from food. The life energy in the body breaks up the foods and converts them into energy also. It is the intricate task of the life force to distil more life force from the nourishment taken into the body. Therefore, one's dietary should be confined to food that are easily converted into energy, or which are productive of fresh energy. Oxygen and sunshine should have a very important place in people's lives, because of their direct energy producing quality. The more you depend on the will and on Cosmic Energy to sustain you, the less your food requirements; the more you depend on food, the weaker your food requirements; the more you depend on food, the weaker your will and the less your recourse to Cosmic Energy.

The magnetic diet consists of such food substitutes as rays and oxygen which can be easily assimilated and converted into energy by the latent life forces in the body. Magnetic foods give energy more quickly than solids and liquids which are less easily converted into life force.

When you are tired or hungry, take a sun bath, and you will find yourself recharged with ultraviolet rays, and revived; or inhale and exhale several times outdoors or near an open window, and your fatigue will be gone. A fasting person who inhales and exhales deeply twelve times, three times a day, recharges his body with electrons and free energy from air and ether. Contact of food and oxygen with the inner bodily system is necessary if the life force is to convert the food and oxygen into energy. The life force can assimilate oxygen more quickly than it can assimilate solids or liquids.

Practice the following exercise three times a day: Exhale slowly, counting from 1 to 6. Now, while the lungs are empty, mentally count from 1 to 6. Inhale slowly, counting from 1 to 6, then hold the breath, counting from 1 to 6. Repeat eleven times.

Just as electricity passes through a rod mad of a conductive substance, and electrifies it, so the body battery becomes fully charged with life force derived from oxygen. People who perform breathing exercises always have shining, magnetic eyes.
One hour's sun bath is also a part of the magnetic diet.

The ultraviolet rays which one absorbs in one whole day on a bathing beach exert a beneficial vitalizing effect on the body, which lasts about three months. Sores and wounds can be cured by exposing them one half hour daily to the sunlight.

Treatment with artificially produced ultraviolet and infrared rays also supplies the body with magnetic nourishment. Much benefit may be derived from it if it is taken under the guidance of a specialist.

Ordinary window glass prevents the sun's ultraviolet rays from penetrating into a room.

Living in a sun room enclosed by yellow quartz glass, through which the ultraviolet sun rays penetrate, would supply the human body with magnetic spiritual nutriment and make it in turn spiritually magnetic. A man living in a room enclosed by red quartz glass would find brute force developing within himself.

Each one of the many billions of cells within the human body is a tiny mouth taking nourishment. The life force, identified with the body, creates within us a desire to derive energy from the circulation and from meat and other foods taken into the stomach. The life force must be trained to draw energy from subtler sources. The body's energy requirements can be supplied partly by sunshine and oxygen, which are absorbed by the pores. For this reason, the surface of the skin must be kept scrupulously clean at all times.

Exercising with will and concentration produces excellent results because it creates energy directly, by will development. This energy is quickly absorbed by the muscles, blood, bones, and sinews, for cellular rejuvenation. Therefore, the highest degree of energy accompanied by the least tissue destruction is derived from the Yogoda will exercises (Lessons 1 to 3).

Occasionally charging the body with electricity by holding on to two electrodes of a battery is a good method for supplying the body with free energy. (The electric current should be very weak.) Bathing in sunlight-heated or ultra-violet-ray-saturated water is very beneficial.

Rubbing the whole stripped body vigorously and rapidly with the palms before taking a bath generates life force and is also very beneficial.

If a weak man wrestles or lives in the same room with a strong, vital individual, he absorbs some of the latter's vital and mental magnetism. For this reason young and old people should mingle and thus exchange magnetism. Different people have different kinds of vitality. Always try to discover new methods for getting direct energy qualities from different individuals.

As a rule, the word "food" is used only in connection with material nourishment, but there are other kinds of food: mental energy, or concentration, and Divine Wisdom. The first (material food) recharges the body battery; the second (concentration), the mind battery; the third (Divine Wisdom), the soul battery.

Not only are proper material foods in the right combinations necessary for the sustenance of the body, but they exert a decided influence on the brain. The spiritual brain, the active brain, and the material brain are all affected by food, and can form different combinations: (1) spiritual active brain, (2) intellectual active brain, and (3) material active brain.

All food that is eaten produces a sensation on the palate as well as certain chemical effects in body and brain. Food sensations determine a specific mentality. Foods such as dried meat produce gross material reactions which develop the material brain and animal mind. Likewise, the eating of active, vital foods, such as onions, garlic, fresh (not dried) meat, etc., produces an active brain. Eating raw fruits and vegetables produces spiritual qualities in the consumer and develops a spiritual mind and brain.

The quality of the food's taste and color is all reported to the brain through the nerves of taste and sight, and is experienced as specific pleasant or unpleasant sensations. These sensations are elaborated into perceptions and conceptions. Repeated conceptions about foods form definite mental habits and manifest themselves as material, active, or spiritual qualities.

While we know that material foods supply the body with energy, we must also remember that good thoughts are nourishing food for the mind, and thoughts of any other nature are poisonous to the health of body and mind.

Have you ever analyzed your magnetic mental diet? It consists usually of the thoughts which you are thinking as well as the thoughts you are receiving from the close thought contact with your friends. Peaceful thoughts and peaceful friends always produce healthy, magnetic minds. It is easy to tell whether a person feeds on a quarrelsome or a peaceful environment. Inner disquietude and worries, due to the wrong sort of friends or unappreciative immediate relatives, produce an unwholesome, gloomy mind.

*Ridding the mind of worry poisons:* If you are suffering from mental ill-health, go on a mental diet. A health-giving mental fast will clear the mind and rid it of the accumulated mental poisons resulting from a careless, faulty mental diet.

First of all, learn to remove the causes of your worries without permitting them to worry you. Do not feed your mind with daily created mental poisons of fresh worries.

Worries are often the result of attempting to do too many things hurriedly. Do not "bolt" your mental duties, but thoroughly masticate them, one at a time, with the teeth of attention and saturate them with the saliva of good judgement. Thus will you avoid worry indigestion.

*Worry fasts.* Then you must go on worry fasts. Three times a day shake off all worries. At seven o'clock in the morning say to yourself, "All my worries of the night are cast out, and from 7 to 8 A.M. I refuse to worry, no matter how troublesome are the duties ahead of me. I am going on a *worry fast.*" From 12 to 1 P.M., say, "I am cheerful, I will not worry."
In the evening, between six and nine o'clock, while in the company of your husband or wife or "hard-to-get-along-with" relatives or friends, mentally make a strong resolution and say, "Within these three hours I will not worry, I refuse to get vexed, even if I am nagged. No matter how tempting it is to indulge in a *worry feast,* I will resist the temptation. I have been very sick of worries – my heart of peace has been diseased. I have had several worry heart attacks. I must not paralyze and kill my peace-heart by shocks of worries. I am on a *worry fast.* I cannot afford to worry."

After you succeed in carrying out *worry fasts* during certain hours of the day, try doing it for a week or two weeks at a time, and then try to prevent the accumulation of worry poisons in your system, entirely.

Whenever you find yourself indulging in a *worry feast,* go on a partial or complete *worry fast* for a day or a week.

Whenever you make up your mind not to worry, *i.e.,* to go on *worry fast, stick to your resolution.* You can stop worrying entirely. You can calmly solve your most difficult problems, putting forth your greatest effort, and at the same time absolutely refuse to worry. Tell your mind, "I can do only my best; no more. I am satisfied and happy that I *am* doing my best to solve my problem; there is absolutely no reason why I should worry myself to death."

When you are on a *worry fast,* you need not be in a negative mental state. Drink copiously of the fresh waters of peace flowing from the spring of every circumstance, vitalized by your determination to be cheerful. If you have made up your mind to be cheerful, nothing can make you unhappy. If you do not choose to destroy your own peace of mind by accepting the suggestion of unhappy circumstances, none can make you dejected. You are concerned only with the untiring performance of right *actions* for right results; but your whole attention must be on the actions, and not on their results. Leave the latter to God, saying, "I have done my best under the circumstances. Therefore, I am happy."

*Joy as a cure for worry:* The negative method for overcoming worry poisoning is *worry fasting.* There are also positive methods. One infected with the germs of worry must go on a strict mental diet. He must feast frugally, but regularly, on the society of joyful minds. Every day he must associate – if only for a little while – with "joy-infected" minds. There are some people the song of whose laughter nothing can still. Seek them out and feast with them on this most vitalizing food of joy. Continue the laughter diet for a month or two. Feast on laughter in the company of really joyful people. Digest it thoroughly by whole-heartedly masticating laughter with the teeth of your attention. Steadfastly continue your laughter diet once you have begun it, and at the end of a month or two you will see the change – your mind will be filled with sunshine. Remember, specific habits can be cultivated only by specific habit-forming actions.

*The courage diet:* Having benefited by the *worry fast,* try the *fear fast* next, going on a courage diet for certain hours, days, or weeks. You must act spiritually in order to be spiritual.

*The wisdom diet:* In order to destroy ignorance, go on *a wisdom diet.* Drink the tonic of wisdom from the lips of intuition. You can learn from intuition when you meet it in the chamber of deep meditation. Read good books of a devotional and spiritual nature, taking from them what you need.

Consult a spiritual specialist. If your disease of ignorance is chronic, be guided entirely by him. That patient cannot be cured who depends only on his own judgment which may be affected by his state of mental ill health.

Go on ignorance-elimination fasts. Refuse to be enslaved by ignorant habits and thoughtless actions. Take up intensive spiritual study and intensive spiritual dieting, and refuse to suffer any longer from the infection of ignorance.

*Overcoming mental stagnation:* Mental stagnation is "mental T.B." Come out of your closed chamber of narrowness. Drink in the fresh air of others' vital thoughts and views. Drink vitality; receive mental nourishment from materially and spiritually progressive minds. Feast unstintingly on the creative thinking within yourself and others. Take long mental walks on the paths of self-confidence. Exercise with the instruments of judgment, introspection, and initiative. Exhale poisonous thoughts of discouragement, discontentment, hopelessness, etc. Inhale the fresh oxygen of success, and know that you are progressing with God's help. This will recharge your soul battery. By consciously destroy mental stagnation and acquire progressive spiritual health and wisdom.

*Acquiring physical, mental and spiritual perfection:* Thus, day by day, eating spiritual magnetism-producing foods and absorbing vitality-producing sunshine, you will physically reflect God's everlasting youth. Eliminating all mental poisons and partaking of the divine nourishment of determination, courage, continuous, unfailing mental effort and concentration, you will learn to overcome the most difficult problems with ease. Eliminating ignorance by constant meditation on God, and following the precepts of Yogoda and your spiritual teacher, you will attain perfect spiritual health. Once you acquire this spiritual health, you will give your life to and for others, to show them also the way to supreme, intoxicating spiritual health.

Once you learn to eat right foods, think right thoughts, being filled with wisdom and joy, your body, mind, and soul will be spiritualized and perceived as dynamos of magnetic energy. Your body and mind, purified by this energy, will take on the beauty of the Spirit. Once you realize yourself as a soul, you will know you are of the Spirit, resting everywhere equally in joy, in all space, in all things, as one with all things.

A body, mind, and soul magnet, recharged with good food, rays, power, wisdom, and Bliss, draws unto itself all material and spiritual souls, spiritually deeply magnetic, like itself. A spiritual magnet is charged with the life of God, and whomsoever it touches, it makes God of him.

## SUMMARY

Those who think that life depends only on breakfast, lunch and dinner – on solids and liquids – are gross-minded. We can derive energy either from material foods or from the Cosmic Source.

The man of the future will draw nourishment from the ether and from the ocean of invisible Cosmic Energy in which he moves and has his being.

It is the aim of this lesson:
    (1) To direct the student's attention to the advisability of drawing his energy requirements, so far as possible, from

air and sunlight. The nourishment derived from these two sources can be most easily converted into energy within the body.

(2) To show the student the necessity of choosing only those material foods which emit and lodge spiritual vibrations in man's mind and brain.

Material foods impress the mind with certain good or bad qualities, and people's thoughts, actions, and health generally are determined by the foods they eat.

## Food and Health Recipes

SWAMI PUDDING

2 ½ slices whole wheat bread (1/2 inch thick)
1 cup seedless raisins
½ cup sugar
3 eggs
½ tsp.vanilla extract
3 ½ large tbsp. butter
Pinch of salt

Remove dark part of crust from bread. Cut bread in ½ in. squares and crisp, but do not scotch, in oven. Add melted butter. Stir bread in it till butter is all soaked up. Place in bottom of pudding dish. Cover with raisins (well washed). Beat eggs, add salt, sugar, vanilla and milk and pour over bread and raisins. Cut tiny pieces of butter over the top of pudding and cook in very slow oven until custard is barely set. Serve with cream, (plain or whipped) and jam or honey.

NOTE: Too long cooking or too hot oven makes the custard tough.

## NUTMEAT LOAF

1 cup English walnuts
1 large potato
1 large onion
1 large carrot
1 cup cooked rice
1 cup milk
½ cup tomato juice
½ cup chili sauce
½ cup chopped parsley
4 tablespoons butter
1 tablespoon curry powder
½ tsp salt

Put nuts, potato, onion and carrot through the food-chopper. Add the rice, milk, tomato juice, chili sauce and the seasonings. Mix well. Turn into a well buttered baking dish and bake one hour in a moderate oven. (350 F).

ORIENTAL DELIGHT
(A Dessert)

Make a soft custard as follows:

3 egg yolks
3 tablespoons sugar
1 pint rich milk
1 tablespoon vanilla extract
1 teaspoon lemon extract

Put yolks into a bowl. Do not beat the yolks. Stir the sugar into them gradually. Heat the milk in a double boiler until boiling. Add it slowly to the egg and sugar. Turn the mixture into the double boiler and cook over a slow fire until the mixture thickens. Stir constantly. Do not allow the milk to boil or it will curdle. When the mixture coats the spoon, it is thick enough. Cool, and add extracts. Chill in refrigerator.

Have ready parfait glasses or other dessert dishes. Put in each glass 3 chopped dates or nuts and some sweet jelly. When ready to serve, fill the glasses with the custard and sprinkle with chopped nuts.

# Mahavatar Babaji

## Chapter 33
## Autobiography of A Yogi

# *Babaji, the Yogi-Christ of Modern India*

The northern Himalayan crags near Badrinarayan are still blessed by the living presence of Babaji, guru of Lahiri Mahasaya. The secluded master has retained his physical form for centuries, perhaps for millenniums. The deathless Babaji is an *avatara.* This Sanskrit word means "descent"; its roots are *ava,* "down," and *tri,* "to pass." In the Hindu scriptures, *avatara* signifies the descent of Divinity into flesh.

"Babaji's spiritual state is beyond human comprehension," Sri Yukteswar explained to me. "The dwarfed vision of men cannot pierce to his transcendental star. One attempts in vain even to picture the avatar's attainment. It is inconceivable."

The *Upanishads* have minutely classified every stage of spiritual advancement. A *siddha* ("perfected being") has progressed from the state of a *jivanmukta* ("freed while living") to that of a *paramukta* ("supremely free"-full power over death); the latter has completely escaped from the mayic thralldom and its reincarnational round. The *paramukta* therefore seldom returns to a physical body; if he does, he is an avatar, a divinely appointed medium of supernal blessings on the world.

An avatar is unsubject to the universal economy; his pure body, visible as a light image, is free from any debt to nature. The casual gaze may see nothing extraordinary in an avatar's form but it casts no shadow nor makes any footprint on the ground. These are outward symbolic proofs of an inward lack of darkness and material bondage. Such a God-man alone knows the Truth behind the relativities of life and death. Omar Khayyam, so grossly misunderstood, sang of this liberated man in his immortal scripture, the *Rubaiyat:*

*"Ah, Moon of my Delight who know'st no wane,*
*The Moon of Heav'n is rising once again;*

297

Mahavatar Babaji

*How oft hereafter rising shall she look*
*Through this same Garden after me-in vain!"*

The "Moon of Delight" is God, eternal Polaris, anachronous never. The "Moon of Heav'n" is the outward cosmos, fettered to the law of periodic recurrence. Its chains had been dissolved forever by the Persian seer through his self-realization. "How oft hereafter rising shall she look . . . after me-in vain!" What frustration of search by a frantic universe for an absolute omission!

Christ expressed his freedom in another way: "And a certain scribe came, and said unto him, Master, I will follow thee whithersoever thou goest. And Jesus saith unto him, The foxes have holes, and the birds of the air have nests; but the Son of man hath not where to lay his head."[1]

Spacious with omnipresence, could Christ indeed be followed except in the overarching Spirit?

Krishna, Rama, Buddha, and Patanjali were among the ancient Indian avatars. A considerable poetic literature in Tamil has grown up around Agastya, a South Indian avatar. He worked many miracles during the centuries preceding and following the Christian era, and is credited with retaining his physical form even to this day.

Babaji's mission in India has been to assist prophets in carrying out their special dispensations. He thus qualifies for the scriptural classification of *Mahavatar* (Great Avatar). He has stated that he gave yoga initiation to Shankara, ancient founder of the Swami Order, and to Kabir, famous medieval saint. His chief nineteenth-century disciple was, as we know, Lahiri Mahasaya, revivalist of the lost *Kriya* art.

The *Mahavatar* is in constant communion with Christ; together they send out vibrations of redemption, and have planned the spiritual technique of salvation for this age. The work of these two fully-illumined masters-one with the body, and one without it-is to inspire the nations to forsake suicidal wars, race hatreds, religious sectarianism, and the boomerang-evils of materialism. Babaji is well aware of the trend of modern times, especially of the influence and complexities of Western civilization, and realizes the necessity of spreading the self-liberations of yoga equally in the West and in the East.

That there is no historical reference to Babaji need not surprise us. The great guru has never openly appeared in any century; the misinterpreting glare of publicity has no place in his millennial plans. Like the Creator, the sole but silent Power, Babaji works in a humble obscurity.

Great prophets like Christ and Krishna come to earth for a specific and spectacular purpose; they depart as soon as it is accomplished. Other avatars, like Babaji, undertake work which is concerned more with the slow evolutionary progress of man during the centuries than with any one outstanding event of history. Such masters always veil themselves from the gross public gaze, and have the power to become invisible at will. For these reasons, and because they generally instruct their disciples to maintain silence about them, a number of towering spiritual figures remain world-unknown. I give in these pages on Babaji merely a hint of his life-only a few facts which he deems it fit and helpful to be publicly imparted.

No limiting facts about Babaji's family or birthplace, dear to the annalist's heart, have ever been discovered. His speech is generally in Hindi, but he converses easily in any language. He has adopted the simple name of Babaji (revered father); other titles of respect given him by Lahiri Mahasaya's disciples are Mahamuni Babaji Maharaj (supreme ecstatic saint), Maha Yogi (greatest of yogis), Trambak Baba and Shiva Baba (titles of avatars of Shiva). Does it matter that we know not the patronymic of an earth-released master?

"Whenever anyone utters with reverence the name of Babaji," Lahiri Mahasaya said, "that devotee attracts an instant spiritual blessing."

The deathless guru bears no marks of age on his body; he appears to be no more than a youth of twenty-five. Fair-skinned, of medium build and height, Babaji's beautiful, strong body radiates a perceptible glow. His eyes are dark, calm, and tender; his long, lustrous hair is copper-colored. A very strange fact is that Babaji bears an extraordinarily exact resemblance to his disciple Lahiri Mahasaya. The similarity is so striking that, in his later years, Lahiri Mahasaya might have passed as the father of the youthful-looking Babaji.

Swami Kebalananda, my saintly Sanskrit tutor, spent some time with Babaji in the Himalayas.

"The peerless master moves with his group from place to place in the mountains," Kebalananda told me. "His small band contains two highly advanced American disciples. After Babaji has been in one locality for some time, he says: *'Dera danda uthao.'* ('Let us lift our camp and staff.') He carries a symbolic *danda* (bamboo staff). His words are the signal for moving with his group instantaneously to another place. He does not always employ this method of astral travel; sometimes he goes on foot from peak to peak.

Babaji can be seen or recognized by others only when he so desires. He is known to have appeared in many slightly different forms to various devotees-sometimes without beard and moustache, and sometimes with them. As his undecaying body requires no food, the master seldom eats. As a social courtesy to visiting disciples, he occasionally accepts fruits, or rice cooked in milk and clarified butter.

"Two amazing incidents of Babaji's life are known to me," Kebalananda went on. "His disciples were sitting one night around a huge fire which was blazing for a sacred Vedic ceremony. The master suddenly seized a burning log and lightly struck the bare shoulder of a chela who was close to the fire.

"Sir, how cruel!" Lahiri Mahasaya, who was present, made this remonstrance.

"Would you rather have seen him burned to ashes before your eyes, according to the decree of his past karma?"

"With these words Babaji placed his healing hand on the chela's disfigured shoulder. 'I have freed you tonight from painful death. The karmic law has been satisfied through your slight suffering by fire.'

"On another occasion Babaji's sacred circle was disturbed by the arrival of a stranger. He had climbed with astonishing skill to the nearly inaccessible ledge near the camp of the master.

"Sir, you must be the great Babaji." The man's face was lit with inexpressible reverence. 'For months I have pursued a ceaseless search for you among these forbidding crags. I implore you to accept me as a disciple.'

"When the great guru made no response, the man pointed to the rocky chasm at his feet.

"If you refuse me, I will jump from this mountain. Life has no further value if I cannot win your guidance to the Divine."

"Jump then," Babaji said unemotionally. 'I cannot accept you in your present state of development.'

The man immediately hurled himself over the cliff. Babaji instructed the shocked disciples to fetch the stranger's body. When they returned with the mangled form, the master placed his divine hand on the dead man. Lo! he opened his eyes and prostrated himself humbly before the omnipotent one.

"You are now ready for discipleship." Babaji beamed lovingly on his resurrected chela. 'You have courageously passed a difficult test. Death shall not touch you again; now you are one of our immortal flock.' Then he spoke his usual words of departure, '*Dera danda uthao*'; the whole group vanished from the mountain."

An avatar lives in the omnipresent Spirit; for him there is no distance inverse to the square. Only one reason, therefore, can motivate Babaji in maintaining his physical form from century to century: the desire to furnish humanity with a concrete example of its own possibilities. Were man never vouchsafed a glimpse of Divinity in the flesh, he would remain oppressed by the heavy mayic delusion that he cannot transcend his mortality.

Jesus knew from the beginning the sequence of his life; he passed through each event not for himself, not from any karmic compulsion, but solely for the upliftment of reflective human beings. His four reporter-disciples-Matthew, Mark, Luke, and John-recorded the ineffable drama for the benefit of later generations.

For Babaji, also, there is no relativity of past, present, future; from the beginning he has known all phases of his life. Yet, accommodating himself to the limited understanding of men, he has played many acts of his divine life in the presence of one or more witnesses. Thus it came about that a disciple of Lahiri Mahasaya was present when Babaji deemed the time to be ripe for him to proclaim the possibility of bodily immortality. He uttered this promise before Ram Gopal Muzumdar, that it might finally become known for the inspiration of other seeking hearts. The great ones speak their words and participate in the seemingly natural course of events, solely for the good of man, even as Christ said: "Father . . . I knew that thou hearest me always: but *because of the people which stand by I said it,* that they may believe that thou hast sent me."[2]

During my visit at Ranbajpur with Ram Gopal, "the sleepless saint,"[3] he related the wondrous story of his first meeting with Babaji.

"I sometimes left my isolated cave to sit at Lahiri Mahasaya's feet in Benares," Ram Gopal told me. "One midnight as I was silently meditating in a group of his disciples, the master made a surprising request.

"Ram Gopal," he said, 'go at once to the Dasasamedh bathing *ghat.*'

I soon reached the secluded spot. The night was bright with moonlight and the glittering stars. After I had sat in patient silence for awhile, my attention was drawn to a huge stone slab near my feet. It rose gradually, revealing an underground cave. As the stone remained balanced in some unknown manner, the draped form of a young and surpassingly lovely woman was levitated from the cave high into the air. Surrounded by a soft halo, she slowly descended in front of me and stood motionless, steeped in an inner state of ecstasy. She finally stirred, and spoke gently.

"I am Mataji,[4] the sister of Babaji. I have asked him and also Lahiri Mahasaya to come to my cave tonight to discuss a matter of great importance."

A nebulous light was rapidly floating over the Ganges; the strange luminescence was reflected in the opaque waters. It approached nearer and nearer until, with a blinding flash, it appeared by the side of Mataji and condensed itself instantly into the human form of Lahiri Mahasaya. He bowed humbly at the feet of the woman saint.

Before I had recovered from my bewilderment, I was further wonder-struck to behold a circling mass of mystical light traveling in the sky. Descending swiftly, the flaming whirlpool neared our group and materialized itself into the body of a beautiful youth who, I understood at once, was Babaji. He looked like Lahiri Mahasaya, the only difference being that Babaji appeared much younger, and had long, bright hair.

"Lahiri Mahasaya, Mataji, and myself knelt at the guru's feet. An ethereal sensation of beatific glory thrilled every fiber of my being as I touched his divine flesh.

"Blessed sister," Babaji said, 'I am intending to shed my form and plunge into the Infinite Current.'

"I have already glimpsed your plan, beloved master. I wanted to discuss it with you tonight. Why should you leave your body?" The glorious woman looked at him beseechingly.

"What is the difference if I wear a visible or invisible wave on the ocean of my Spirit?"

Mataji replied with a quaint flash of wit. 'Deathless guru, if it makes no difference, then please do not ever relinquish your form.'[5]

"Be it so," Babaji said solemnly. 'I will never leave my physical body. It will always remain visible to at least a small number of people on this earth. The Lord has spoken His own wish through your lips.'

As I listened in awe to the conversation between these exalted beings, the great guru turned to me with a benign gesture.
"Fear not, Ram Gopal," he said, 'you are blessed to be a witness at the scene of this immortal promise.'

As the sweet melody of Babaji's voice faded away, his form and that of Lahiri Mahasaya slowly levitated and moved backward over the Ganges. An aureole of dazzling light templed their bodies as they vanished into the night sky. Mataji's form floated to the cave and descended; the stone slab closed of itself, as if working on an invisible leverage.

"Infinitely inspired, I wended my way back to Lahiri Mahasaya's place. As I bowed before him in the early dawn, my guru smiled at me understandingly."

"I am happy for you, Ram Gopal," he said. 'The desire of meeting Babaji and Mataji, which you have often expressed to me, has found at last a sacred fulfillment.'

"My fellow disciples informed me that Lahiri Mahasaya had not moved from his dais since early the preceding evening.

"He gave a wonderful discourse on immortality after you had left for the Dasasamedh *ghat*," one of the chelas told me. For the first time I fully realized the truth in the scriptural verses which state that a man of self-realization can appear at different places in two or more bodies at the same time.

"Lahiri Mahasaya later explained to me many metaphysical points concerning the hidden divine plan for this earth," Ram Gopal concluded. "Babaji has been chosen by God to remain in his body for the duration of this particular world cycle. Ages shall come and go-still the deathless master,[6] beholding the drama of the centuries, shall be present on this stage terrestrial."

---

[1] Matthew 8:19-20.

[2] John 11:41-42.

[3] The omnipresent yogi who observed that I failed to bow before the Tarakeswar shrine (chapter 13).

[4] "Holy Mother." Mataji also has lived through the centuries; she is almost as far advanced spiritually as her brother. She remains in ecstasy in a hidden underground cave near the Dasasamedh ghat.

[5] This incident reminds one of Thales. The great Greek philosopher taught that there was no difference between life and death. "Why, then," inquired a critic, "do you not die?" "Because," answered Thales, "it makes no difference."

# The Science of Kriya Yoga

Chapter 26
Autobiography of a Yogi

The science of *Kriya Yoga,* mentioned so often in these pages, became widely known in modern India through the instrumentality of Lahiri Mahasaya, my guru's guru. The Sanskrit root of *Kriya* is *kri,* to do, to act and react; the same root is found in the word *karma,* the natural principle of cause and effect. *Kriya Yoga* is thus "union (yoga) with the Infinite through a certain action or rite." A yogi who faithfully follows its technique is gradually freed from karma or the universal chain of causation.

Because of certain ancient yogic injunctions, I cannot give a full explanation of *Kriya Yoga* in the pages of a book intended for the general public. The actual technique must be learned from a *Kriyaban* or *Kriya Yogi;* here a broad reference must suffice.

*Kriya Yoga* is a simple, psychophysiological method by which the human blood is decarbonized and recharged with oxygen. The atoms of this extra oxygen are transmuted into life current to rejuvenate the brain and spinal centers. [1] By stopping the accumulation of venous blood, the yogi is able to lessen or prevent the decay of tissues; the advanced yogi transmutes his cells into pure energy. Elijah, Jesus, Kabir and other prophets were past masters in the use of *Kriya* or a similar technique, by which they caused their bodies to dematerialize at will.

*Kriya* is an ancient science. Lahiri Mahasaya received it from his guru, Babaji, who rediscovered and clarified the technique after it had been lost in the Dark Ages.

"The *Kriya Yoga* which I am giving to the world through you in this nineteenth century," Babaji told Lahiri Mahasaya, "is a revival of the same science which Krishna gave, millenniums ago, to Arjuna, and which was later known to Patanjali, and to Christ, St. John, St. Paul, and other disciples."

*Kriya Yoga* is referred to by Krishna, India's greatest prophet, in a stanza of the *Bhagavad Gita:* "Offering inhaling breath into the outgoing breath, and offering the outgoing breath into the inhaling breath, the yogi neutralizes both these breaths; he thus releases the life force from the heart and brings it under his control." [2] The interpretation is: "The yogi arrests decay in the body by an addition of life force, and arrests the mutations of growth in the body by *apan* (eliminating current). Thus neutralizing decay and growth, by quieting the heart, the yogi learns life control."

Krishna also relates[3] that it was he, in a former incarnation, who communicated the indestructible yoga to an ancient illuminato, Vivasvat, who gave it to Manu, the great legislator.[4] He, in turn, instructed Ikshwaku, the father of India's solar warrior dynasty. Passing thus from one to another, the royal yoga was guarded by the rishis until the coming of the materialistic ages.[5] Then, due to priestly secrecy and man's indifference, the sacred knowledge gradually became inaccessible.

*Kriya Yoga* is mentioned twice by the ancient sage Patanjali, foremost exponent of yoga, who wrote: "*Kriya Yoga* consists of body discipline, mental control, and meditating on *Aum.*"[6] Patanjali speaks of God as the actual Cosmic Sound of *Aum* heard in meditation.[7] *Aum* is the Creative Word,[8] the sound of the Vibratory Motor. Even the yoga-beginner soon inwardly hears the wondrous sound of *Aum.* Receiving this blissful spiritual encouragement, the devotee becomes assured that he is in actual touch with divine realms.

Patanjali refers a second time to the life-control or *Kriya* technique thus: "Liberation can be accomplished by that *pranayama* which is attained by disjoining the course of inspiration and expiration."[9] St. Paul knew *Kriya Yoga,* or a technique very similar to it, by which he could switch life currents to and from the senses. He was therefore able to say: "Verily, I protest by our rejoicing which I have in Christ, *I die daily.*" [10] By daily withdrawing his bodily life force, he united it by yoga union with the rejoicing (eternal bliss) of the Christ consciousness. In that felicitous state, he was consciously aware of being dead to the delusive sensory world of *maya.*

In the initial states of God-contact (*sabikalpa samadhi*) the devotee's consciousness merges with the Cosmic Spirit; his life force is withdrawn from the body, which appears "dead," or motionless and rigid. The yogi is fully aware of his bodily condition of suspended animation. As he progresses to higher spiritual states (*nirbikalpa samadhi*), however, he communes with God without bodily fixation, and in his ordinary waking consciousness, even in the midst of exacting worldly duties.[11]

"*Kriya Yoga* is an instrument through which human evolution can be quickened," Sri Yukteswar explained to his students. "The ancient yogis discovered that the secret of cosmic consciousness is intimately linked with breath mastery. This is India's unique and deathless contribution to the world's treasury of knowledge. The life force, which is ordinarily absorbed in maintaining the heart-pump, must be freed for higher activities by a method of calming and stilling the ceaseless demands of the breath."

The *Kriya Yogi* mentally directs his life energy to revolve, upward and downward, around the six spinal centers (medullary, cervical, dorsal, lumbar, sacral, and coccygeal plexuses) which correspond to the twelve astral signs of the zodiac, the symbolic Cosmic Man. One-half minute of revolution of energy around the sensitive spinal cord of man effects subtle progress in his evolution; that half-minute of *Kriya* equals one year of natural spiritual unfoldment.

The astral system of a human being, with six (twelve by polarity) inner constellations revolving around the sun of the omniscient spiritual eye, is interrelated with the physical sun and the twelve zodiacal signs. All men are thus affected by an inner and an outer universe. The ancient rishis discovered that man's earthly and heavenly environment, in twelve-year cycles, push him forward on his natural path. The scriptures aver that man requires a million years of normal, diseaseless evolution to perfect his human brain sufficiently to express cosmic consciousness.

One thousand *Kriya* practiced in eight hours gives the yogi, in one day, the equivalent of one thousand years of natural evolution: 365,000 years of evolution in one year. In three years, a *Kriya Yogi* can thus accomplish by intelligent self-effort the same result which nature brings to pass in a million years. The *Kriya* short cut, of course, can be taken only by deeply developed yogis. With the guidance of a guru, such yogis have carefully prepared their bodies and brains to receive the power created by intensive practice.

The *Kriya* beginner employs his yogic exercise only fourteen to twenty-eight times, twice daily. A number of yogis achieve emancipation in six or twelve or twenty-four or forty-eight years. A yogi who dies before achieving full realization carries with him the good karma of his past *Kriya* effort; in his new life he is harmoniously propelled toward his Infinite Goal.

The body of the average man is like a fifty-watt lamp, which cannot accommodate the billion watts of power roused by an excessive practice of *Kriya.* Through gradual and regular increase of the simple and "foolproof" methods of *Kriya,* man's body becomes astrally transformed day by day, and is finally fitted to express the infinite potentials of cosmic energy-the first materially active expression of Spirit.

*Kriya Yoga* has nothing in common with the unscientific breathing exercises taught by a number of misguided zealots. Their attempts to forcibly hold breath in the lungs is not only unnatural but decidedly unpleasant. *Kriya,* on the other hand, is accompanied from the very beginning by an accession of peace, and by soothing sensations of regenerative effect in the spine.

The ancient yogic technique converts the breath into mind. By spiritual advancement, one is able to cognize the breath as an act of mind-a dream-breath.

Many illustrations could be given of the mathematical relationship between man's respiratory rate and the variations in his states of consciousness. A person whose attention is wholly engrossed, as in following some closely knit intellectual argument, or in attempting some delicate or difficult physical feat, automatically breathes very slowly. Fixity of attention depends on slow breathing; quick or uneven breaths are an inevitable accompaniment of harmful emotional states: fear, lust, anger. The restless monkey breathes at the rate of 32 times a minute, in contrast to man's average of 18 times. The elephant, tortoise, snake and other animals noted for their longevity have a respiratory rate which is less than man's. The tortoise, for instance, who may attain the age of 300 years,[12] breathes only 4 times per minute.

The rejuvenating effects of sleep are due to man's temporary unawareness of body and breathing. The sleeping man becomes a yogi; each night he unconsciously performs the yogic rite of releasing himself from bodily identification, and of merging the life force with healing currents in the main brain region and the six sub-dynamos of his spinal centers. The sleeper thus dips unknowingly into the reservoir of cosmic energy which sustains all life.

The voluntary yogi performs a simple, natural process consciously, not unconsciously like the slow-paced sleeper. The *Kriya Yogi* uses his technique to saturate and feed all his physical cells with undecaying light and keep them in a magnetized state. He scientifically makes breath unnecessary, without producing the states of subconscious sleep or unconsciousness.

By *Kriya,* the outgoing life force is not wasted and abused in the senses, but constrained to reunite with subtler spinal energies. By such reinforcement of life, the yogi's body and brain cells are electrified with the spiritual elixir. Thus he removes himself from studied observance of natural laws, which can only take him-by circuitous means as given by proper food, sunlight, and harmonious thoughts-to a million-year Goal. It needs twelve years of normal healthful living to effect even slight perceptible change in brain structure, and a million solar returns are exacted to sufficiently refine the cerebral tenement for manifestation of cosmic consciousness.

Untying the cord of breath which binds the soul to the body, *Kriya* serves to prolong life and enlarge the consciousness to infinity. The yoga method overcomes the tug of war between the mind and the matter-bound senses, and frees the devotee to reinherit his eternal kingdom. He knows his real nature is bound neither by physical encasement nor by breath, symbol of the mortal enslavement to air, to nature's elemental compulsions.

Introspection, or "sitting in the silence," is an unscientific way of trying to force apart the mind and senses, tied together by the life force. The contemplative mind, attempting its return to divinity, is constantly dragged back toward the senses by the life currents. *Kriya,* controlling the mind *directly* through the life force, is the easiest, most effective, and most scientific avenue of approach to the Infinite. In contrast to the slow, uncertain "bullock cart" theological path to God, *Kriya* may justly be called the "airplane" route.

The yogic science is based on an empirical consideration of all forms of concentration and meditation exercises. Yoga enables the devotee to switch off or on, at will, life current from the five sense telephones of sight, sound, smell, taste, and touch. Attaining this power of sense-disconnection, the yogi finds it simple to unite his mind at will with divine realms or with the world of matter. No longer is he unwillingly brought back by the life force to the mundane sphere of rowdy sensations and restless thoughts. Master of his body and mind, the *Kriya Yogi* ultimately achieves victory over the "last enemy," death.
*So shalt thou feed on Death, that feeds on men:*
*And Death once dead, there's no more dying then.*[13]

The life of an advanced *Kriya Yogi* is influenced, not by effects of past actions, but solely by directions from the soul. The devotee thus avoids the slow, evolutionary monitors of egoistic actions, good and bad, of common life, cumbrous and snail-like to the eagle hearts.

The superior method of soul living frees the yogi who, shorn of his ego-prison, tastes the deep air of omnipresence. The thralldom of natural living is, in contrast, set in a pace humiliating. Conforming his life to the evolutionary order, a man can command no concessionary haste from nature but, living without error against the laws of his physical and mental endowment, still requires about a million years of incarnating masquerades to know final emancipation.

The telescopic methods of yogis, disengaging themselves from physical and mental identifications in favor of soul-individuality, thus commend themselves to those who eye with revolt a thousand thousand years. This numerical periphery is enlarged for the ordinary man, who lives in harmony not even with nature, let alone his soul, but pursues instead unnatural complexities, thus offending in his body and thoughts the sweet sanities of nature. For him, two times a million years can scarce suffice for liberation.

Gross man seldom or never realizes that his body is a kingdom, governed by Emperor Soul on the throne of the cranium, with subsidiary regents in the six spinal centers or spheres of consciousness. This theocracy extends over a throng of obedient subjects: twenty-seven thousand billion cells-endowed with a sure if automatic intelligence by which they perform all duties of bodily growths, transformations, and dissolutions-and fifty million substratal thoughts, emotions, and variations of alternating phases in man's consciousness in an average life of sixty years. Any apparent insurrection of bodily or cerebral cells toward Emperor Soul, manifesting as disease or depression, is due to no disloyalty among the humble citizens, but to past or present misuse by man of his individuality or free will, given to him simultaneous with a soul, and revocable never.

Identifying himself with a shallow ego, man takes for granted that it is he who thinks, wills, feels, digests meals, and keeps himself alive, never admitting through reflection (only a little would suffice!) that in his ordinary life he is naught but a puppet of past actions (karma) and of nature or environment. Each man's intellectual reactions, feelings, moods, and habits are circumscribed by effects of past causes, whether of this or a prior life. Lofty above such influences, however, is his regal soul. Spurning the transitory truths and freedoms, the *Kriya Yogi* passes beyond all disillusionment into his unfettered Being. All scriptures declare man to be not a corruptible body, but a living soul; by *Kriya* he is given a method to prove the scriptural truth.

"Outward ritual cannot destroy ignorance, because they are not mutually contradictory," wrote Shankara in his famous *Century of Verses.* "Realized knowledge alone destroys ignorance. . . . Knowledge cannot spring up by any other means than inquiry. 'Who am I? How was this universe born? Who is its maker? What is its material cause?' This is the kind of inquiry referred to." The intellect has no answer for these questions; hence the rishis evolved yoga as the technique of spiritual inquiry.

*Kriya Yoga* is the real "fire rite" often extolled in the *Bhagavad Gita.* The purifying fires of yoga bring eternal illumination, and thus differ much from outward and little-effective religious fire ceremonies, where perception of truth is oft burnt, to solemn chanted accompaniment, along with the incense!

The advanced yogi, withholding all his mind, will, and feeling from false identification with bodily desires, uniting his mind with superconscious forces in the spinal shrines, thus lives in this world as God hath planned, not impelled by impulses from the past nor by new witlessnesses of fresh human motivations. Such a yogi receives fulfillment of his Supreme Desire, safe in the final haven of inexhaustibly blissful Spirit.

The yogi offers his labyrinthine human longings to a monotheistic bonfire dedicated to the unparalleled God. This is indeed the true yogic fire ceremony, in which all past and present desires are fuel consumed by love divine. The Ultimate Flame receives the sacrifice of all human madness, and man is pure of dross. His bones stripped of all desirous flesh, his karmic skeleton bleached in the antiseptic suns of wisdom, he is clean at last, inoffensive before man and Maker.

Referring to yoga's sure and methodical efficacy, Lord Krishna praises the technological yogi in the following words: "The yogi is greater than body-disciplining ascetics, greater even than the followers of the path of wisdom (*Jnana Yoga*), or of the path of action (*Karma Yoga*); be thou, O disciple Arjuna, a yogi!"[14]

---

[1] The noted scientist, Dr. George W. Crile of Cleveland, explained before a 1940 meeting of the American Association for the Advancement of Science the experiments by which he had proved that all bodily tissues are electrically negative, except the brain and nervous system tissues which remain electrically positive because they take up revivifying oxygen at a more rapid rate

.

[2] Bhagavad Gita, IV:29.

[3] Ibid. IV:1-2.

[4] The author of Manava Dharma Shastras. These institutes of canonized common law are effective in India to this day. The French scholar, Louis Jacolliot, writes that the date of Manu "is lost in the night of the ante-historical period of India; and no scholar has dared to refuse him the title of the most ancient lawgiver in the world." In La Bible dans l'Inde, pages 33-37, Jacolliot reproduces parallel textual references to prove that the Roman Code of Justinian follows closely the Laws of Manu.

[5] The start of the materialistic ages, according to Hindu scriptural reckonings, was 3102 B.C. This was the beginning of the Descending Dwapara Age (see page 174). Modern scholars, blithely believing that 10,000 years ago all

men were sunk in a barbarous Stone Age, summarily dismiss as "myths" all records and traditions of very ancient civilizations in India, China, Egypt, and other lands.

[6] Patanjali's Aphorisms, II:1. In using the words Kriya Yoga, Patanjali was referring to either the exact technique taught by Babaji, or one very similar to it. That it was a definite technique of life control is proved by Patanjali's Aphorism II:49.

[7] Ibid. I:27.

[8] "In the beginning was the Word, and the Word was with God, and the Word was God. . . . All things were made by him; and without him was not any thing made that was made."-John 1:1-3. Aum (Om) of the Vedas became the sacred word Amin of the Moslems, Hum of the Tibetans, and Amen of the Christians (its meaning in Hebrew being sure, faithful). "These things saith the Amen, the faithful and true witness, the beginning of the creation of God."-Revelations 3:14.

[9] Aphorisms II:49.

[10] I Corinthians 15:31. "Our rejoicing" is the correct translation; not, as usually given, "your rejoicing." St. Paul was referring to the omnipresence of the Christ consciousness.

[11] Kalpa means time or aeon. Sabikalpa means subject to time or change; some link with prakriti or matter remains. Nirbikalpa means timeless, changeless; this is the highest state of samadhi.

[12] According to the Lincoln Library of Essential Information, p. 1030, the giant tortoise lives between 200 and 300 years.

[13] Shakespeare: Sonnet #146.

[14] Bhagavad Gita, VI:46.

# Yogavatar Shama Lahiri Mahasaya's Ladder

Excerpt from article
Inner Culture
March, 1937

In contradistinction to most prophets, Lahiri Mahasaya did not try to inspire people with improved doctrines. He showed them the step-by-step methods of Self-Realization, by which truth-thirsty people would redeem themselves by properly living them in life and bring out the ignorance-shrouded image of God into distinct human consciousness.

## Hastening Evolution

Sunlight and food change the human body, brain and mind every seven years (there is a twelve-year cycle also), provided there is no physical sickness. It takes one million solar years to evolve the healthy human body, brain and mind so that they are able to manifest Cosmic Consciousness.

Since the human body cannot last so long, Lahiri Mahasaya devised the Kriya technique which so changes brain-cells, spine and body that they can express Cosmic Consciousness in three, six or twelve years (in determined, advanced students) and in twenty-four to forty-eight years (in ordinary students.)

Christ gave techniques of salvation to St. John and the disciples, promising to send to them the Comforter, about which people understand little.

Lahiri Mahasaya's teaching is the Second Coming of Christ, not through a mere claim, but in actuality. His Kriya technique of meditation expands the cup of concentration so that it can be large enough to hold the ocean of Christ-consciousness, (consciousness that was present in the life of Jesus.) Lahiri Mahasaya's technique can reveal to each soul that God belongs to him by divine birthright and has not to be evolutionarily attained. But actual step-by-step meditation is necessary in order to destroy self-created delusion. The prodigal son walked away from God. *Each of his retracing footsteps back to God consists of a mental technique which enables him to return.*

318

## Praying Unceasingly

Jesus Christ spoke of praying unceasingly or with ever-increasing concentration until God was realized. Do most of the modern Christians try to meditate as Jesus commanded? Most of them pray for a little while, with an automobile ride or a chicken dinner remaining in the background of their minds.

Christ spoke of Holy Ghost or Great Sacred Ghostlike Invisible Intelligent Cosmic Vibration which is responsible for creation of all solid, liquid, gaseous and energy substances.

In the beginning of the creation of finite things like solids, liquids, gases and energy substances was the Word (the combination of Cosmic Vibration and Cosmic Intelligence) and God is the Word or Intelligent Cosmic Vibration. Science agrees with this fact, that Intelligent Cosmic Vibration differentiates itself into an ordered creation of solids, liquids, gases, etc.

This Cosmic Vibration manifests as Cosmic Light, Cosmic Sound and Cosmic Ever-New Joy of which St. John speaks: "I was in the Spirit (God contact) and heard (realized thru intuition) behind me the voice of a great trumpet (Cosmic Sound)."

## The Comforter

Lahiri Mahasaya's Kriya technique is the fulfillment of Jesus Christ's promise to send the Comforter. Through Kriya the devotee can expand his consciousness from the body to infinity, without losing consciousness, by tuning in with the actual Cosmic Sound or the Holy Ghost sound emanating form the vibration of all atoms and electrons. When the devotee tunes himself with this sound, he finds the greatest all-sorrow-quenching Comfort and perceives his Spirit present not only in his little body but in all vibrating space.

Patanjali speaks of listening to this Cosmic Om. Science knows that there is a Cosmic Hum emanating from all atoms. St. John says, "I heard behind me….. a great trumpet." Lahiri Mahasaya speaks of tuning and expanding the soul into Cosmic Vibration. All Christians and truth-seekers need not believe forever what Lahiri Mahasaya taught, but need to believe only for the purpose of demonstrating the truth of the teachings in their own Self-Realization.

After the passing of a prophet, his inspiration usually is changed into a dogmatic creed by his blind adherents, but the followers of Lahiri Mahasaya are given step-by-step wonderful methods of meditation which work and which yield results of ever-increasing divine joy from the beginning, if practiced intensely. Therefore, Self-Realization of Divine Bliss-contact of God and not beliefs holds the followers of Self-Realization Fellowship together.

Hence Christians and all truth seekers who have suffered long from theological indigestion ought to try Lahiri Mahasaya's world-emancipating technique with scientific steadiness, just as they might join a university, and find for themselves that God can be contacted in this life, *now*.

The life of Lahiri Mahasaya set an example which changed the erroneous notion that yoga is a mysterious practise.

Every man may find a way through Kriya to understand his proper relation with nature and to feel spiritual reverence for all phenomena, whether mystical or everyday occurences, in spite of the matter-of-factness of physical sicence.

The Law of Kriya Yoga is eternal. It is like mathematics, like the simple rules of addition and subtraction, the law of Kriya can never be destroyed. Burn to ashes all the books on Mathematics, the logically-minded will always rediscover such truths, destroy all the sacred books on yoga, its fundamental laws will come out whenever there appears a true yogi who comprises within himself pure devotion and consequently pure knowledge.

# More books from Alight Publications

## Breathe Like Your Life Depends On It
Author: *Rudra Shivananda*
Explore the secrets of Life-force control and expansion for self-Healing, strength and vitality. Imagine living a life protected from stress and ill-health, with wisdom and strength. This is the fruit of controlling and expanding the life-force energy called *prana.* Powerful, simple and beneficial practices which utilize the life-force in the breath, to rejuvenate the body and transform our emotional, mental and spiritual being.
[ 208 pages. US$18.5]

## *Chakra* selfHealing by the power of *OM*
Author: *Rudra Shivananda*
A practical workbook on healing and spiritual evolution. Tap into the potential of the primary energy centers of the body, to eliminate depression and fatigue, relieve anxiety and stress, and calm the mind to achieve inner happiness. Learn the effective *yogic* system of tuning, balancing, color healing, rejuvenation, emotional detoxification, energization, and transcendence, with the *chakras,* in a simple, and step-by-step practice.
[140 pages. US$15.0]

## Dew-Drops of the Soul
Author: *Yogiraj Gurunath*
A unique compilation of poetic gems from a contemporary Himalayan Master, expressing the essence of his inner experience, as a guide and inspiration for all spiritual seekers.
[ 106 pages. US$12.5]

## Earth Peace through Self Peace
Author: *Yogiraj Gurunath*
A collection of spiritual talks or *satsangs*, answering the questions from sincere seekers of truth. A Master speaks to the soul through the doorway of the heart, opening the reader to the reality of the true Self, in spite of the limitations of human language. *Yogiraj* speaks from his own direct experience, in his own simple, direct way, clearing away all doubts and irrelevancies.
[164 pages. US$16.5]

## Surya Yoga
Author: *Rudra Shivananda*

Tap into the awesome, everpresent healing power of our life-giving Sun. Through the sincere and constant practice of the *Surya Sadhana* [solar practice], you will heal the physical body, acquire greater vitality, overcome all negativity, and also come to a greater understanding and realization of your true nature. Illustrated step-by-step instructions. [164 pages, US$16.5]

## Time and the Human Condition
Author: *Partap Singh*

An examination of time, perspective, and our ability to understand, will reveal steps we can take to solve some of the more vexing problems of the modern world. To help us to take the first steps to better understand ourselves and the world around us, the author sheds light on the nature of time through the limited but sharp lens of science, how our views of the afterlife affect our conduct in this life, how limited perspective affect education, government, and justice and how our sense of time affect our attitudes on stress and love. [ 220 pages,  $13.5]

## Wings to Freedom
Author: *Yogiraj Gurunath Siddhanath*

Mystic Revelations fom the immortal Babaji and other Himalayan Yogis, as experienced by a perfected Master, Yogiraj Gurunath Siddhanath. Follow his footsteps and experience through his words, as he walks his talk in the jungles, temples, ashrams and hidden [to the uninitiated] places of India. Enrich your life with the secret oral traditions revealed for the first time - mysteries of life, immortality and the attainment of Self-Realization.
[308 pages, US$22.5]

## Yoga of Purification and Transformation
Author: *Rudra Shivananda*

Attain Peace of Mind in this life and Terminate the cycle of suffering caused by the accumulation of negative karma. Learn the 5 yogic restrainsts or yamas which constitute the Yoga of Purification and the 5 yogic observances or niyamas which are the heart of the Yoga of Transformation. An inspiring and informative presentation of the often neglected foundation of all successful spiritual practice. Actual detailed practices are given in addition to relevant examples and parables. [220 pages, US$18.5]

*For information on these or other books or to purchase them
on-line with credit card, visit our web-site:
htttp://www.alightbooks.com*

CPSIA information can be obtained
at www.ICGtesting.com
Printed in the USA
BVHW071202090819
555497BV00001B/47/P